THE RELENTLESS PURSUIT OF YOU

THE RELENTLESS PURSUIT OF YOU

SIX PILLARS TO TAKE BACK YOUR LIFE

SHAWN RIDER

Praise for *The Relentless Pursuit of You*

"The perfect balance between a slap in the face and a hug."
-**Colm O'Reilly**, Owner, CrossFit Ireland

"A raw, no nonsense kick in the ass to get your life right, and get on with an amazing life NOW, NO EXCUSES! Teaching college for over 20 years, I have always told my students that there is more to life than your job and chasing the dollar. This book reinforces that concept, but also provides individuals with a real world road map of what they can do to build a life using fundamental pillars of strength. Save the cost of a life coach or counselor, and just pick up and read this book!"
-**Herb Brown, Ph.D.**, Professor of Workforce Leadership & Development and Business, Marketing & Entrepreneurship Education at Appalachian State University

"Shawn illustrates logical and sequential steps to building the 'you,' you desire."
-**Kent Houchins**, COO, Grafton Integrated Health Network

"Shawn is to the point. He'll have you laughing and crying all in the same chapter. If you've ever questioned how to go about reaching your goals, and want a practical, honest approach to doing it, this book is a must read."
-**Nadine Pottinga**, President/CEO, United Way of Northern Shenandoah Valley

"Wow. After reading The Relentless Pursuit of You, *I was able to recognize that I was putting too much effort into some pillars and not enough into others. Shawn does a great job teaching people how to fix their shit, rather than just saying 'fix your shit.'"*
-**Ron White**, Owner, CrossFit Tried and True

Praise for *The Relentless Pursuit of You*

"Shawn does a phenomenal job at delivering a graceful reality check. Take ownership of these six pillars in your life and you will absolutely celebrate the victories of your decision to relentlessly pursue a better you."
-**Daniel Fritsch**, Assistant Chief of Operations, Fire and Rescue Department

"As an English teacher, I believe in the power of words to motivate and inspire people. Many authors of personal development books aim to do just that, but fall remarkably short. They tell us what we need to change and why we need to change those things, but very rarely do they explain HOW to do it, leaving the reader unfulfilled, and frankly, wondering whether it was worth the cost. In The Relentless Pursuit of You, *Shawn Rider provides the reader with a blunt, yet accessible account of not only the what and why, but also the HOW: a toolbox of methods to help you fix your shit and keep it fixed, which, at the end of the day, is priceless."*
-**Crystal Gage**, AP English Teacher, John Handley High School

"Shawn Rider tells us what we need to hear, not necessarily what we want to hear. But because he is a coach through and through, The Relentless Pursuit of You *always reads as empathetic, as cajoling, and as supportive. This is a book that will appeal to those who are familiar with self-improvement and those who are taking their first bite at the apple. There are practical nuggets interspersed with big, overarching themes, but it's the insistent reminders of truths that you already know in your heart that make the explosive impact. Shawn is here to make sure you know the power that small adjustments, relentlessly pursued, can have on your health, your relationships, and your happiness."*
-**Ari Sommer**, Esquire and Member, Harrison & Johnston, PLC

"This book should be required reading for anyone who is looking to live their best life, and isn't afraid to constantly move forward in personal growth."
-**Stuart Brauer**, Owner, WTF Gym Talk

The Relentless Pursuit of You:
Six Pillars to Take Back Your Life
Copyright © 2019 SHAWN RIDER

All rights reserved. No part of this book may be reproduced or transmitted in any form or by any means, electronic or mechanical, including photocopying, recording, or by any information storage and retrieval system, without written permission from the author, except for the inclusion of brief quotations in a review.

Disclaimer: While the publisher and author have used their best efforts in preparing this book, they make no representations or warranties with respect to the accuracy or completeness of the contents of this book and specifically disclaim any implied warranties of merchantability or fitness for a particular purpose. No warranty may be created or extended by a sales representative or written sales materials. The advice and strategies contained herein may not be suitable for your situation. You should consult with a professional where appropriate. Neither the publisher, nor author shall be liable for any loss or profit, or any other personal or commercial damages, including, but not limited to: special, incidental, consequential, or other damages.

Author: Shawn Rider
Editor: Crystal Gage
Cover Design: Greg Scriot, Greg Scriot's Imagine and Create

Print ISBN 9781798939949

To your relentless pursuit of _____.

Please, feel free to post your dedication page and any part of this book, including your challenges, to Instagram and tag @therelentlesspursuitofyou with #therelentlesspursuitofyou

You can also follow the author @shawn_rider_ on Instagram

CONTENTS

1	**Introduction**	9
2	**The Pillars**	17
3	**Exercise**	28
4	**Food**	35
5	**Sleep**	50
6	**Personal Development**	61
7	**Stressors / Media**	84
8	**Connection**	103
9	**The Catalyst**	129
10	**Journal**	161
	Acknowledgements	170
	References	172

1 | INTRODUCTION

We've become too comfortable. The alarm goes off at the same time every day. Breakfast never changes, if we eat it at all. We leave for work at the same time, and drive the same route every morning. At work, we have the same routine: clock in, punch a few keys, sign a few papers, and clock out. And then, every night, we eat an unbalanced dinner, watch the same shows, and pack the same damn bag to start all over again the next day.

But that's not the problem.

We all have daily, repeatable tasks, but we've now put our entire lives on autopilot. Both our bodies and minds are on repeat. For many, as soon as they wake up, the main goal is to get to the end of the day. I'm an advocate of structure, organization, routine, and consistency, but only when they are pulling me toward a better version of myself. This can only occur if I am upholding the six essential pillars that support physical and mental growth, all of which are outlined in this book. Any routine that does not allow a person to grow is unfavorable.

That's the problem.

==Routine can be beneficial, but only if it's giving you the ability to truly thrive from day to day.== Are you optimizing the time you have every day, or are you stuck on the treadmill going five miles per hour, watching the same old news channel as life passes you by?

You may have a positive and steady workout routine that starts at five every morning, yet you lack a results-driven eating plan. You're so accustomed to putting cream and way too much sugar in your coffee that you can't even imagine your morning cup of joe without them. And what's worse is that you know excessive sugar consumption is bad for you, but again, you're too comfortable, so you haven't tried to change. You are neglecting a pillar that is essential to reaching your goals.

. . . . .

When I was a high school teacher, the goal of many of my colleagues was to survive until the final bell rang, barely skating by for 30 days, and getting their paychecks on the last day of the month; then, they would start that cycle all over again. And it wasn't just the teachers. It was also the administrators. They'd put out fire after fire (mostly petty disciplinary issues and parental complaints that prevented them from ever stepping foot into a positive learning environment), and then they'd do it again the next day. There was no real leadership or ownership for the progress, or lack thereof, being made in our school system. Most teachers and administrators made no forward or meaningful progress in their professional development throughout the entire year, or worse, multiple years.

I believe that if you're not making progress in your own life, you can't help or encourage others (your children, spouses, co-workers, friends) to progress in theirs. Everything in your life starts with you. Remember, there is a huge difference between surviving daily and thriving daily.

. . . . .

This never ending daily cycle of survival isn't living at all. Being stuck in such a cycle slowly destroys your body, your mind, and ultimately, your life. I don't want that type of life for you. That is why I'm writing this book. You aren't supposed to just survive. You should optimize. You should thrive. You should not just live, you should LIVE. No matter what has happened, no matter what your past decisions have been, you can reignite your life. You accomplish this by relentlessly pursuing a better life, and a better version of yourself.

Therefore, the goal I have for you is to allow the pillars outlined in this book to help you thrive, every day, relentlessly, for the rest of your life.

· · · · ·

When you were a child, who did you hope to become? Have you stopped chasing that person? Who have you actually become? As long as you're reading this book, it's safe to say that you're still alive, and that means you have the time and the ability to change. You can decide what you want for your life, and who you want to become. Who or what are you chasing for yourself? "No one" or "nothing" should never be the answer.

You'll notice throughout this book that I ask questions and make statements that will make you stop and really ponder your own answer, or even make you frustrated in disagreement. Good. I want you to question your own motives. Questioning your own motives creates inner dialogue and conflict which produces a better opportunity for you to grow than inner criticism does. You should never stop asking how you can improve. You should be unrelenting in the journey to better yourself.

Also, while reading this book, you might realize that you have one pillar pretty well taken care of, but what about another? Find your weak pillar and believe that you can strengthen it. You not only can, but you must, solidify the foundations of your life.

But why? Why even try?

Because you are a freaking human being, and life is precious, but short. So, each of the pillars will improve your life, not only for your current self, but also your future self.

. . . . .

As a gym owner, I work with several clients who have specific goals for their physical fitness, whether that means losing weight, or getting stronger, or both. I will present you with the same challenge I present to each of them: you must imagine that every decision you make requires a negotiation between your current self (the self who requires improvements in some regard) and your future, ideal self (the self who has achieved the goals set forth by your current self). Your current self is a byproduct of negotiations from your past, negotiations that may have resulted in choosing an option that was counterproductive to the goals you saw for yourself in the future. For example, if you are overweight, it's because you've made countless negotiations between eating healthy foods or unhealthy foods, and most of those negotiations resulted in eating the unhealthy foods. Even if some of them ended in eating healthy foods, at the end of the day, majority rules, and your body reacts accordingly, applying the results of those negotiations to your future self. But because these negotiations are entirely internal conflicts, you have the final say in terms of every single one of them, and therefore, you have the power to change the trend that your current self has created. The fact is that if you ever want to meet the future self you envision in your mind, the person who has improved his/her life and reached some pretty incredible goals, you have to learn how to negotiate according to those standards. From this point forward, you're not making decisions for the person you currently are; you're doing it for the person you want to meet a year from now.

No matter what stage you're at in your life (college graduate, new parent, single dad, unemployed, business owner, grandparent), you are allowed to improve your life. You are allowed to alter the path you've been taking to chase the person you have always wanted to become. I'm going to venture to say that it's not so much that you're allowed to change, but that you should change. When we say someone has changed, it tends to carry a negative connotation. But if we truly reflect on why we add cynicism to that statement, it's usually because the people we are discussing have taken control of an aspect of their lives and made it better. Because of that, their values no longer align with ours, and we get mad that they have taken the initiative that we can't seem to take ourselves. If someone comes up to me and says that I've changed, my response is to smile and say, "Thank you." In ten years, you shouldn't be the same person you are today. The question is, will you be better or worse off because of the decisions you're making today?

· · · · ·

I'm an optimistic realist. Every person has the ability to define success on his/her own terms, and then use that definition to become successful. That's the optimist in me. But as I look out onto the landscape of society, realism slaps me in the face. As a gym owner, it's my job to hold the metaphorical mirror up in front of clients and show them what their current actions or inactions have given them. Being a realist compels me to make sure they know the state of their current situations, whether it's good or bad. We can't start a journey or know where we want to go until we truly know where we are right now. Then, I need to show them that they can reach their desired goals. Being optimistic about the future, while at the same time being a realist about this moment in time is step number one in taking back your life. Step number two is consistently building and maintaining the pillars that provide the foundations for personal progress.

2 | THE PILLARS

Taking back your life begins with prioritizing pillars that will allow you to be healthy, energized, recovered, and ready to handle what happens around you on a daily basis.

You can't reach any long term goal for yourself, your family, your career, or your business if you don't know how these pillars fit into your life, or how you're going to prioritize them on a regular basis.

There are six pillars.

Three are labeled as external: activities that require the use of and provide benefit to your body.

Three are labeled as internal: activities that require the use of and provide benefit to your mind.

Each pillar has both external and internal benefits, though. On some level, all six require you to make both a conscious (internal) decision and an active (external) decision, which means all of the pillars benefit you in your totality.

The six pillars are:

1. **Exercise** (external)
2. **Food** (external)
3. **Sleep** (external)
4. **Personal Development** (internal)
5. **Stressors / Media** (internal)
6. **Connection** (internal)

You may be dialed in on some of these pillars, but completely missing the others.

Example: you may work out every single day (exercise), have a growing and positive relationship (connection), and are a part of a great team at work (connection) that puts an emphasis on continuing education in your field of expertise (personal development). But at the same time, from Monday through Friday you go to bed way too late (sleep), eat out with coworkers for lunch (food), and if you looked at your phone's usage, the weekly average would be the equivalent of an entire day of full-time work (stressors/media). You have pillars that are falling down or missing entirely. What happens to a structure if the supports are weak or deteriorating? It crumbles. Although these pillars can fall apart over time if no attention is paid to them, they can also be rebuilt.

Maybe the above describes your lifestyle. Maybe it doesn't. Chapter 10 will provide you with a journal that starts with a time audit, and it will show you where your priorities currently lie regarding each pillar. But we aren't there yet.

. . . . .

Before you move on and hear my spiel about the pillars over the next few chapters, I must first clarify an important concept of this book. If you don't first believe that it's possible for you to be relentless in the pursuit of a better you, and if your mind is not open to learning, implementing, and executing the strategies that will help you do so, you might as well just put this book down and walk away. Don't waste your time.

But if you have come to the realization that you've done nothing more than accept the current state of your life over the past few years, whether it is good or bad, and you want to push past those self-imposed limitations, then you need this book. In order for this book to be worth the money you've spent and the time you'll invest in reading it, action must prevail. If these pages motivate you, great. But motivation isn't the long term purpose of this book. Consistent, persistent, relentless action is the holy grail you are seeking.

You can change. You can improve, revamp, or tweak all six pillars. ==Don't reach for or expect perfection, but acknowledge that you can consistently do better.== Taking a misstep, forgetting something, or even failing happens, and that is okay. ==What is not okay is calling yourself a failure and giving up.==

In 2006, Carol Dweck, Ph. D., published her breakthrough book, *Mindset: The New Psychology of Success,* which is based on her numerous years of studying how and why people view and respond to success and failure differently. She found that there are two types of mindsets people can have: a fixed mindset or a growth mindset. I won't get into the nitty-gritty details. You can read the book, and I most certainly recommend that you do, but basically, people with fixed mindsets believe they cannot improve their current abilities, intelligence, or learn new skills. Their traits are fixed, and their success and failure relies solely on their innate abilities. In other words, they cannot improve in a particular area if they don't already possess a high level of skill in that area. On the other hand, ==people with growth mindsets believe that they can improve and positively impact their abilities, intelligence, and even learn new skills if they work hard==

and focus on improving over the long run. Growth oriented people use obstacles as motivation to push forward and improve. People with fixed mindsets are more prone to give up when facing obstacles, and do only what naturally comes easy to them.

In her book, Dweck quotes an article from *The New York Times* that stated, *"failure has been transformed from an action (I failed) to an identity (I am a failure). This is especially true in the fixed mindset."* Failure, the action ("I failed"), can be a good thing if you learn from it. Failure, the identity ("I am a failure"), is always a bad thing. Learn and remember the difference.

If you've tried to eat better, but after a few weeks you had a piece of chocolate cake and told yourself you weren't "cut out for this" and "can't do this," you have a fixed mindset toward eating better. If you consistently went to the gym for a month, but then your trainer made you do something you struggled with, so you never went back, you have a fixed mindset toward exercise. If you read those two examples and immediately thought, "Yup! That's me! I have a fixed mindset! So hell, thanks for telling me that. I shouldn't even get started," you have a fixed mindset toward personal growth. I need you to read the next sentence slowly.

You. Can. Change. Your. Mindset.

Again, but a little louder for the people in the back.

==You. Can. Change. Your. Mindset.==

•   •   •   •   •

I'm grateful that for most of my life, I've had a growth mindset that has allowed me to work through my failures. But looking back, there was a point when I had a fixed mindset.

Growing up, football was my sport, my main thing. I played from fourth grade until my sophomore year in college. In my junior and senior years of high school, I suffered season ending injuries during the first game of each season. I was the captain of our team. I had hopes to play on a scholarship at an NCAA Division I school. So, needless to say, these injuries were devastating for me and my family. Not one college coach called me after hearing I had been injured.

Wanting to prove that I could still play for an elite school, I walked on (meaning I didn't have a scholarship, but still tried out for the team) at Appalachian State University, a college that had just won its second straight Division I-AA (now called Division I FCS) National

Championship. Two weeks after graduating high school, I moved from Hanover, PA to Boone, NC to train with the football team and start my college courses instead of "celebrating" my final summer before college. At the end of the summer, I made the team. This was one of my greatest achievements, a goal accomplished by using a growth mindset.

But, unfortunately, after earning a position on the team, and eventually being offered a spot in the preseason fall camp during my sophomore year (colleges can only take a certain percentage of players for the fall camp, so this was another goal achieved), I fell into a fixed mindset. I started looking at how fast the other players were compared to me. I saw how much they could bench and squat compared to me. I saw the scholarship players, who were now three-star recruits due to AppState winning its third national title in a row during my freshman year, getting preferential treatment (I mean, the schools were paying for them to be there, so why wouldn't they get the first shot at everything, right?). I started to believe that no matter how much effort I put in, I wasn't meant to play football at that level. Couple that with another injury in fall camp (dislocated knee cap), and that was the straw that broke the camel's back. I quit playing football after that season ended.

For the two months following the end of my football career, I did nothing but sleep, go to class, go to the gym, study, and watch TV. In other words, in my mind, there was nothing to strive toward. That is, until my thoughts started to transition back into a growth mindset. Instead of using that growth mindset for sports, however, I started applying it to my grades in school. I remember taking the first quiz in my introductory accounting class the semester immediately after quitting football. I got an F on the quiz, but instead of devastating me, it motivated me to do better. A few weeks later, we had our first test. The accounting department at AppState took its tests pretty seriously, so every professor gave the same test at the same time to all of the students in accounting courses for the semester. All 300+ students had to show up on a Friday night at 5 p.m. to take the test during the same three hour time slot.

The next week, our professor came into class and said the average score on the test was a high C. She also stated that out of the 300+ students, only four received perfect scores.

I was one of the four.

· · · · ·

Fast forward a few years from age 20 to 26. My full-time job was as a teacher at a local high school, but I also co-owned a gym that was experiencing enough success that I thought I could eventually leave my teaching career permanently. My business partner was a great guy, but as the gym grew, our goals for the future of the business became different. I admit that I was a terrible communicator at that point in my life. When I didn't get my way or received push back on my opinions, my emotions got the best of me. After a full year of struggle and disagreement, we dissolved the partnership.

Right before the dissolution, we had 72 members. Afterward, there were 9 who decided to keep me as their trainer.

9… out of 72 people.

12.5% of our members stayed with me.

That's the equivalent of a really, really, really bad grade.

A few days after the old gym closed, I had a new one up and running. Nine clients, two classes a day, and no coaches besides me. One morning, my girlfriend at the time (now my wife), walked in on me crying on the bedroom floor. I spouted off a few comments about how I couldn't believe this happened. How long would it take for this new gym to grow to the point of being able to earn a livable wage? How much money would it take? How could I ever leave teaching now? Should I just focus on being a teacher? Blah, blah, blah.

But after that Niagara Falls cry session, I got my ass off of the floor and went back to work the next day. Thankfully, my growth mindset was stronger than my fixed mindset.

As I sit here today typing this book, I am filled with gratitude that in that moment, during that season of my life, I allowed myself to acknowledge the failure of my first gym, but, at the same time, did not allow the action of failing to define me as a failure.

· · · · ·

Right now, you may view yourself as a failure. You may have allowed past failings to stop you from accomplishing more in life. You may have stopped taking action. The failures from your past aren't why you are where you are; your inaction after those failures are why you are where you are. You cannot relentlessly pursue something while standing still. You cannot have goals, dreams, or wishes, whatever you want to call them, and then sit idly watching another day, week, month, year, and, soon enough, decade pass you by. The same goes for people who have succeeded. Their inactions or actions after they reach their definition of success is what will determine whether they stay there or not. ==You cannot simultaneously be successful and inactive.== In order for action to take place, you need to be ready to put forth an effort, exert yourself more than ever, and move past your excuses as to why you have been inactive for so long.

Theodore Roosevelt, considered one of the most charismatic Presidents of the United States, once said, *"I always had a horror of words that are not translated into deeds, of speech that does not result in action."* He believed in ==*"realizable ideals and in realizing them, in preaching what can be practiced, and then in practicing it."*==

In December of 2017, I told myself that in 2018 I would write a book. I did not write one page. In December of 2018, I told myself that in 2019 I would write a book.

This is that book.

But the words you're about to read don't mean anything if they don't get you to take action.

3 | EXERCISE

As soon as you wake up in the morning, you check your phone while continuing to lay in bed. After finally getting up, you go to work and likely sit for 8+ hours. And then, you are "so tired" once you get home that you sit for 4+ more hours. This is not what your body is made to do.

==Your body is built to move.==

Imagine getting an Australian Cattle Dog, a dog that was made to work, and penning him up all day, every day. He wouldn't be too happy. He wouldn't listen to you because he'd be chomping at the bit. You are the same way. You're restricting your body from getting what it needs: exercise. And it will punish you if you deprive it of that.

I'm not going to list the health benefits of exercise here. I'm also not going to bash your "I don't have time in my busy schedule" excuse. ==Deep down, we both know that if you prioritized exercise in your life, you'd find the time to do it just like you find the time to lay in bed and stare at your phone each morning.==

What I am going to do is tell you that exercise is much simpler and less intimidating than you think.

Here's the prescription: move your body, elevate your heart rate, and break a sweat a minimum of five days per week. But also understand that if you have particular goals in mind for yourself, you won't achieve them at the local $10/month gym, mimicking the people who are mindlessly walking on a treadmill. Most of those people don't know what they're doing (even if they look like it). I applaud anyone who is at least doing the bare minimum when it comes to exercising, but I'm going to be fully transparent here: if you want to look a certain way, you need to do certain things. If you look at the people who do nothing but walk on treadmills, I'm going to venture a guess that you don't actually want your body to look like that. If you're not sure how to get the results you want, hire a professional: a person who is a certified fitness specialist and earns his/her living helping people exercise. It's 2019! Now more than ever, there are competitively priced options when it comes to getting the individualized support you need to be a healthier you.

In the grand scheme of things, the amount of time you will spend on daily exercise is barely even notable, but yielding results from that small amount of time takes long term dedication and consistency that you may not have had in the last five to twenty years, or maybe ever.

If you work late into the afternoon, work out first thing in the morning.

If you need to be on the road early in the morning, work out in the evening, but ==make sure you're moving your body during the first twenty minutes of the day== (get out of bed and do what your 4th grade physical education teacher made you do: neck circles, arm circles, hip circles, toe touches, etc.).

==Thirty to sixty minutes of exercise a day.== That's all the exercise you need in order to be on the road to good health. However, you have to make that time a priority in your day; the later chapters of this book will help you with that.

. . . . .

I'm biased. I own a "micro gym" called Shenandoah.Fit (also a registered CrossFit affiliate). Our gym strives to keep active memberships under two hundred clients so we can provide quality instruction and education to every active member. We focus on private coaching and group classes ranging from fifteen to twenty people. Group classes are sixty minute sessions which include an instructional warm up tailored specifically for the movements of the day, followed by a high intensity workout ranging from five to thirty minutes. Every member is instructed by a professional coach, whether it's one on one, or in the group model. No one who comes to our gym is left to his/her own devices when it comes to what kind of movements to perform or how to do them, ever.

I personally believe that a group training model in which a client is coached on a regular basis in a supportive environment with like-minded people yields the best possible results for the majority of the population. However, I'm not going to turn this book into a sales pitch for CrossFit[1].

My suggestion is to search for all of the gyms in your area that run organized group classes led by certified coaches. Email or call all of them. Creep on their social media pages and get a feel for how they acknowledge the accomplishments of their current members. Visit each one and see which facility makes YOU feel the most comfortable while you are there. Watch how their current members interact with each other, and more importantly, how their staff interacts with members. Are people smiling? Does it look like they are genuinely enjoying themselves? Exercise should push you past your comfort zone, but you also need to enjoy the atmosphere of the

---

[1] Visit www.crossfit.com for more information on daily workouts and where to find a locally certified gym in your area.

facility and your experience as a whole. Otherwise, you won't return. ==You need to find a place where you want to be each day.==

· · · · ·

With that said, if you do decide to start CrossFit, or any group training program that you've never tried before, my recommendation is that you actually sandbag the crap out of it for at least the first three months.

Why would I suggest such a thing? Because I want you to be safe. I want you to purposely take it slow. I want you to listen and learn from the coaches. I don't want you to get caught up in the intensity and speed of how classes can be run. I don't want you to start comparing yourself to those in class who look like they are killing it, but two years prior were starting from scratch just like you. I want you to enjoy the journey one day and one workout at a time. I want you to feel sore, but not to the point that you're in severe pain. Give your body time to adjust to your new workout routine. If you overwhelm yourself and burn out at the beginning, your exercise journey will be very short, and you will be right back to square one in five months. A private coach can help you establish the right routine.

I want what is best for you. The ultimate goal is to get off of the couch. Walk. Jog. Run. Lift. Stretch. Sweat.

Do it safely, and do it consistently. But no matter what you choose to do for exercise, remember this: just because your fitness journey doesn't look like someone else's, doesn't mean yours is unimportant. It's you versus you, for you.

· · · · ·

Maybe you currently exercise consistently, enjoy the program you're using, and love the results you've gotten. Perfect! Keep going! Use this chapter as a reminder to uphold the pillar of exercise throughout your daily routine.

But maybe you've read this chapter and thought to yourself, "Okay, but I already exercise daily, and the results have been underwhelming." Fair enough. There are probably two main reasons why you aren't seeing progress:

1. Your workout regimen is not tailored to your fitness goals, and you need to hire a professional to create a new one for you.
2. Your nutrition sucks.

With that being said, I have nothing else to add to the exercise pillar, so let's acknowledge the elephant in the room for most people: food.

Chapter Notes

Three Big Takeaways

1.

2.

3.

What do you currently do for exercise?

Do you currently view this pillar as a strength or a weakness?

___

What would you like to accomplish in regard to this pillar over the next 90 days?

12 months?

Are you committed? Can you do this?
P.S. The answer is, "Yes."

4 | FOOD

I believe exercise should be a non-negotiable due to the immediate gratification and positive effects it provides to your body; however, it was only listed as the first pillar because of its sex appeal, not because it's the most important.

Food, on the other hand, is not sexy at all. But, what you eat is King, the Queen Bee, the base of the pyramid (and I'm not referring to the lackluster USDA Food Guide Pyramid). Food is the most important aspect of getting your body to look, feel, and perform the way you want it to.

Food is not fun to talk about with anyone. It doesn't matter if you're talking to a certified professional or someone who has no clue what he/she is doing in terms of nutrition. It's not an enjoyable topic to discuss because 99.9% of people have a food pillar that is just barely standing upright. It's been pulverized by their excuses and the fact that they don't like to be told what they can't or shouldn't eat. When I sit down with a new client at our gym and ask how his/her nutrition is, I always receive the same answer: "Oh, it's pretty good." I've heard that same phrase come out of the mouths of people whose body fat ranges from ten to forty, and, yes, even fifty percent. When a 450 pound man looks you dead in the eye and says his nutrition is "pretty good," you realize that society has been duped.

==We have been deceived, but we also need to take personal responsibility and understand that we have allowed ourselves to become ignorant to the basics of proper nutrition.== Here is a funny, yet serious, example. This past Christmas my mom got me a chocolate bar with almonds in it because "it was the healthy version." All the new trends in dieting say that almonds are a superfood, so adding them to chocolate must make the chocolate a superfood, too. Right? Wrong.

Food is the most effective and important tool for improving your health, both internally and externally, but the information available regarding nutrition is overwhelming. Internet and TV advertisements have led people to believe that there is a magic vegetable shake or special detox that will somehow get them to their goal weights in just fourteen days. Or worse, they believe there is a pill or belly wrap that will reverse all of the horrible food choices they have made for themselves over the course of the last year. And if people actually want to attempt to eat the appropriate foods to lose weight, they think they have to spend exorbitant amounts of money and use incredibly complicated recipes. It's actually easier and more cost effective than you think. Unfortunately, people don't like to hear the cold, hard truth: if you want to see results, you need to consistently eat real, whole foods for the rest of your life.

. . . . .

There are too many "diets." We need to remove the word from the American lexicon. You cannot "diet" for the rest of your life. If you have weight goals, then you should eat according to those goals. Period. If you want to lose weight, you need to eat accordingly, at a caloric deficit. If you want to maintain weight, you need to eat accordingly, at a neutral caloric intake. If you want to gain weight, you need to eat accordingly, at a caloric surplus.

Eat accordingly? Yes. Eat according to your goals. If you want to lose weight, you shouldn't be shoving a store bought apple pie in your face on a Tuesday night, Jim. If you want to drop a pant size by summer, you shouldn't drink half of a bottle of wine before bed because your boss yelled at you on Wednesday, Susan.

"Okay, Shawn. A little aggressive, but I get it. Eat according to my goals. Cool. So, what should I eat?"

I thought you'd never ask. Here are the same four better eating guidelines we give every client at our gym:

1. *Eat whole foods.*
2. *Eat more vegetables.*
3. *Drink water.*
4. *Eat when you're hungry; stop when you're satisfied.*

"Oh, I eat whole foods... the whole pizza! And last week I put lettuce and tomato on my Whopper."

And you probably ordered a Diet Coke to go along with it, didn't you, Bill? Now isn't the time to crack jokes.

"How much water? And can I squirt a little flavor yum-yum in it? Oh, and I'm always hungry and never satisfied!"

Just drink water, Pam. More water. Only water. You should actually hear yourself talk right now. Get control of yourself.

Okay. I got all of the jokes I hear about the above guidelines out of the way. Now I can explain each one as simply as possible, no scientific jargon needed.

Eat whole foods. Whole foods are pretty much anything that was alive or came from the Earth. They are rich in valuable nutrients. Chicken, vegetables, raw nuts, and fruits: yes. Cinnamon Toast Crunch: no.

Eat more vegetables. Fill your plate with vegetables, first. Then, add your chicken breast along with a healthy fat, such as raw nuts or an avocado. Change the type of vegetables you eat daily. A good strategy is to eat a bunch of different colored vegetables. Cycle through the following on a daily basis for good variety: kale, carrots, mixed peppers, onions, asparagus, cauliflower, broccoli, cabbage, etc.

Drink water. A clean, ice-cold glass of water is delicious, especially after a solid workout. Try it sometime. Skip all of the drinks marketed to you as being "vital" post workout recovery drinks. Your average sports drink can have upward of thirty-five grams of sugar. That is the equivalent of a soda. You wouldn't wreck your hard work at the gym by "rehydrating" with a Mountain Dew, so why would you do it with a Gatorade?

Eat when you're hungry; stop when you're satisfied. This last guideline is a little tricky. I absolutely hate the feeling of hunger. I have never "gone hungry," so I shouldn't even say that I hate the feeling. But, once you get your eating under control and establish a better routine (not the "I eat ice cream before bed because I always do" routine… yes, that was my reason back in the day), the feeling of hunger serves a purpose. When you get in tune with your body, it will let you know when it's time to eat. If you're eating whole foods and you eat slowly, you will be satisfied after one well balanced plate. The micronutrients from a variety of vegetables and healthy fats will help you feel fuller, longer. Processed carbohydrates and sugar found in most boxed or bagged foods have the opposite effect.

.　.　.　.　.

Greg Glassman, the founder of CrossFit, Inc., has another simplified, yet powerful prescription for the food we should eat:

"Eat meat and vegetables, nuts and seeds, some fruit, little starch and no sugar. Keep intake to levels that will support exercise but not body fat."

The quality of food comes first. Glassman's quote makes that point very clear and simple for us. The quantity of food comes in at a close second.

Eat whole foods, and cut out as much, if not all, of the processed food you eat regularly. You'll see incredible results. That does not mean you need to skip breakfast and eat a salad with nothing on it for lunch. From my experience as a certified coach and gym owner, undereating the right quality and quantity of healthy foods is just as much an epidemic as overeating unhealthy foods. Start adding in more of the healthy stuff. Once you start doing that, you will naturally start eating less of the unhealthy stuff. It's not about going cold turkey, or labeling foods as "off limits" or "bad." Just start eating legitimately healthy foods listed in the guidelines of this chapter and in Glassman's quote. With that being said, however, if you have specific goals and want to see real change, you also have to be aggressive.

. . . . .

People are too passive in their pursuits of bettering themselves. I guess I should say they are relentlessly too passive in pursuing better lives for themselves. This statement rings no more true than when it comes to cleaning up your eating. You might read this book, immediately drive down to the local globo gym, sign up for a $10/month membership with $1 down, and boom! Tomorrow you'll be there strutting away on the treadmill (#respect if you do that). But if I told you to go into your pantry and throw away everything that is in a box or bag, you'd freak out and start rattling off a bunch of excuses as to why you can't.

Why is that?

Because we've become too passive in regard to wanting to eat better. We've become too dependent on the easy to grab, easy to cook foods. You're scared and nervous to attempt to change those habits due to your past "failings," and that is fueling your passivity.

You need to be aggressive. You need to be assertive and bold in taking this step toward prioritizing healthier foods. If you only buy real, whole foods, you will only eat real, whole foods.

People are a lot quicker when it comes to getting off of the couch than they are getting off of the processed carbohydrates. In their *New York Times* bestselling book *Extreme Ownership: How U.S. Navy SEALs Lead and Win*, Jocko Willink and Leif Babin clarify that "*aggressive means to be proactive.*" Some of you are aggressive with the exercise pillar, yet passive with the food pillar. You may need to shift a little energy from one pillar to the other.

If you're wondering if you're the passive type, then answer this: do you reward yourself with a "treat" after a workout? If the answer is yes, then you're being passive about your nutrition. You're not a dog, so don't give yourself a treat for being a "good boy." Throughout the last six years of owning a gym, our coaches have worked with over ten thousand people, most of whom were seeking to lose body weight, or more specifically, body fat. I can safely say that of those ten thousand people, none of them were already eating healthy foods when they initially sought our help. Let me rephrase that. Not a single person who came to our gym feeling out of shape or overweight could say they got that way by eating whole foods. That person might still be out there, but I have yet to meet anyone who gained fat by eating grilled chicken breast, steamed broccoli, and a small side of sweet potatoes for every meal. It just does not happen.

· · · · ·

Time and money. Those are the two most frequently used excuses when it comes to eating poorly. Yet, with a little brainstorming, neither one has to be a barrier on your path toward better nutrition.

When I was growing up, my family would order take-out every Friday or Saturday night, sometimes both, to the tune of $30+ per meal. Then, early the next week, my parents would complain about finances. Now, as an adult, I can see that healthy food was not a priority in our household, and our finances showed it. I think it's safe to say that this is the case for the average American household. If you look at your bank statement, you'll see where your financial priorities lie. How many restaurants do you see listed? How much of that money could be used to buy quality foods instead? If your goal is to eat healthier foods, then you need to rework your budget to achieve that goal.

If lack of time is the reason you're not eating better, and you absolutely cannot rearrange anything else in your schedule, then it would be beneficial for you to look into local companies that prepare and deliver healthy meals according to your preferences. Can that get expensive? It depends. But if you can't make the time, then you have to spend the money. You can't use both as excuses. Depending on where you are, you could find locally sourced meals for anywhere from $6 to $10, which is typically equivalent to what people spend on a meal when the office orders lunch every day (I've seen clients of mine spend $12 on a Tuesday lunch, then tell me they can't afford our local chef, who sells meals for $5.50 each). Don't be one of those people who says, "I can't spend money on XYZ," and then spends more money on XYZ just because it's packaged differently. If you want to utilize a meal prep company, and lunch is where your nutrition tends to lapse, then only buy enough meals to cover your lunches. If dinner is your problem, and you tend to grab the easy, yet unhealthy, processed carbohydrates, then only buy five meals a week to cover dinner.

· · · · ·

Unfortunately, our beautiful country has sensationalized food. But the thing is, food doesn't have to be sexy. It doesn't have to be some grand, planned out meal. If a company has to market to you what its food's "health" components are, don't eat its food. I've never seen a label that lists ingredients on a bunch of broccoli heads or a locally sourced chicken breast. And don't forget, the big food conglomerates do NOT care that you are trying to lose 20 pounds. Actually, they do not care about you at all. They want you to become addicted to their sugar-packed foods. They don't care about your goals, only your money. They want you to revert back to eating what's easy: the food they put in a box or bag. They spend hundreds of billions of dollars to get you to fail. They hire English majors to write the words that you'll find most attractive, and then make your beloved celebrities say them so that you'll be tricked into thinking you're eating something healthy. I'm getting fired up just typing this paragraph. If someone tries to trick me, if someone doesn't care about my well-being, that is not someone I want to be associated with, and in this case, not a company I want to give my hard-earned money to! Stop paying them to help you fail. Just stop it.

Reread that last paragraph, but this time do it out loud, and take your voice up a few notches. Hell. To. The. Yes! My heart is pumping now.

. . . . .

Finally, eating doesn't need to be an event. It's okay to eat boring food. Not every meal has to be an entirely new eating experience.

It's okay to eat something you don't necessarily enjoy. For me, that something was salmon. Yuck. But I knew it was good for me, so I started eating it for two or three meals each week. Lo and behold, I now like salmon and order it at restaurants.

It's okay to NOT eat the freaking cupcakes Barbara brought to the office for Rick's birthday.

It's okay to pack your own lunch and not order out with your co-workers every Monday, Wednesday, and Friday. Eating out at work is a money pit. If your office is paying for it, may I suggest ordering the salmon and steamed broccoli?

It's okay to shop on the outside of the grocery store and eat as little as possible from boxes and bags. If the container has a cartoon mascot slapped across the front, don't buy it.

You've heard all of this before, but ==now it's time to follow through.==

. . . . .

There are 8 billion people on this planet, and if you get frustrated by "blanket statements" (generalized statements that insinuate fact in all contexts), then you should put this book down. I cannot, nor will I try to, make a detailed eating plan for every person and every possible situation that someone may find him/herself in. I am well aware that the life of a 35 year old, career-oriented, single mom is vastly different than that of a 24 year old, recent college graduate, who goes to the gym twice a day and splits rent with three roommates. I'm also not trying to be the "bad food police." I eat ice cream. I eat the chocolate chip cookies my wife and I bake with our daughter. I can house a whole pizza on a Saturday afternoon. But I also have a pretty good grasp on my food and exercise pillars, so I know when I can indulge in such things without them negatively impacting my body or mind. I don't penalize myself for eating those items every once in a while. Just because I say I can eat them, doesn't mean I always do. But when I do, I don't call it cheating, nor do I punish myself with a harder workout the next day. I just go on to the next day.

A vitally critical aspect in this relentless pursuit of you is realizing which of your pillars are stable. Even more critical, however, is figuring out which ones have crumbled entirely, and how you are going to rebuild them within the confines of your personal schedule and lifestyle. You will have a better grasp of this concept once you complete the exercises in Chapter 10.

I'm not going to go any deeper into the food pillar. If you need guidance, accountability, or any more education regarding your nutrition, seek a professional. Find someone who promotes eating templates and not any one specific diet. If at any point you need a refresher, just reread the four better eating guidelines in this chapter, along with Greg Glassman's quote. Those two pointers will serve you well[2].

P.S. If you find a high quality, well established micro gym, its staff should include qualified individuals who can help you with nutrition. If they do NOT prioritize nutrition inside of their facility, you should NOT be at that facility.

---

[2] I am not a registered dietician or nutritionist. I do not have a degree in the field, nor am I certified to give nutritional or meal plan guidance. If you have any health related problems, you should seek professional guidance.

Chapter Notes

Three Big Takeaways

1.

2.

3.

What do you currently eat most often? Do you cook it or order it?

Do you currently view this pillar as a strength or a weakness?

What would you like to accomplish in regard to this pillar over the next 90 days?

12 months?

Are you committed? Can you do this?
P.S. The answer is, "Yes."

5 | SLEEP

Skipping this chapter would not be in your best interest. Sleep is vitally important. (Insert mind blown and eye roll emoji here.) A quick Google search of "the benefits of sleep" will refresh your memory concerning the significance of this often overlooked task of rest, recovery, and rebuilding.

My goal for you in regard to sleep is twofold:

1. To recognize if you have established an unacceptable routine of deprioritizing your sleep by staying up too late.
2. To learn how to slow your body and mind down before going to sleep, instead of stimulating them.

You are not a teenager anymore. Maybe back in the day you were able to stay up all night playing video games and watching WWE (like my brothers and I used to do). Then, you could wake up for school at 7 a.m., knowing you'd be able to sneak in a nap during Miss Smith's lesson on FDR's New Deal. But that was then, and this is now. Try taking a late afternoon nap in the office when your boss is peacocking around, checking up on the productivity of his workforce, or while your kids are screaming for snacks as they come running into the house after school. It's not going to happen, Sally.

So, when are you supposed to sleep? Well, preferably at night, the way humans have done it for the last 200,000 years. Even though it's 2019, and we live in a society in which work always needs to be done, deadlines are plenty, and bright electronics are constantly in our faces, our bodies are still made to rise and fall with the sun.

. . . . .

Messing with your circadian rhythm by constantly trying to keep yourself awake or energized longer is like incessantly putting your phone on and off of the charger. Every time you get to 53%, you freak out and find the nearest outlet. It's preferred to let your phone's battery, and your body, drain completely before you recharge it to 100%. Quality, uninterrupted sleep in the comfiest bed you can invest in is your body's metaphorical electrical outlet.

So far in this book, you have learned about two pillars that you can more or less start repairing immediately. You can make the conscious decision to go to the gym after work today, or eat a healthy meal for dinner, but when dealing with sleep, your consciousness has no say. Your internal clock will need time to adjust. However, you might find that increasing focus on some of the other pillars will speed up that process. Once it becomes a daily routine for you to exercise, eat whole foods, avoid sugary snacks before bed, read calming literature, cuddle with your partner, and stay off of social media, then POOF! At bedtime, you'll be out like Jose Aldo at the hands of Conor McGregor.

・　　・　　・　　・　　・

What is keeping you up so late?

My wife and I had our first daughter a year ago, so if you're in the new parent phase, have a sleepless child, or a child who needs special attention, I understand. If you work night shift, all of this talk about sleeping at night may come off as useless jargon. In such cases, you can still benefit from these suggestions to better help you sleep during the day.

For the majority of us, lack of sleep, bad quality of sleep, or insufficient time dedicated to sleep is the result of our own doing.

Your actions from the moment you start making dinner until the time you lay in bed are the main determinants of whether or not you'll fall asleep quickly and have quality rest throughout your various sleep cycles.

For example, if you want to sleep well throughout the night, why the heck would you drink a cup of coffee with dinner? At the latest, you should stop drinking caffeine by 2 p.m. There is a time and place for the jitter juice, but in the afternoon, just prior to landing your plane softly for the evening, isn't one of them[3]. Caffeine has a five to six hour half life on average, meaning that after about six hours, half of the caffeine is still in your system. Caffeine affects everyone differently. It can get you so hyped up that you are bouncing off the walls for hours, or, if you're like me, you can drink it before bed and go right to sleep. With that being said, just because you can go to sleep, doesn't mean you're sleeping well. Whether it's a nice cup of hot java or the newest, brightly colored energy in a can, you truly do not need it to get past that mid afternoon crash.

Caffeine should be utilized only after you've been up and moving for thirty minutes, or in the late morning once you have hit your workflow for the day. Only in America do we need an energy drink or a constant flow of coffee in the breakroom to just sit at a desk all day. You get all jacked up just to blankly stare at a computer screen and pound a few keys. Awesome idea, Jim.

---

[3] More recently, I've turned to black or green tea in the afternoon for minimal caffeine intake.

Along the same lines, if you're drinking too much of anything late in the day, you're probably going to need to use the restroom in the middle of the night. However, if you front-load your day with proper hydration, you can afford to start cutting back your liquids after 2 p.m. As soon as I get out of bed, usually around 5:30 a.m., I fill a shaker bottle with 16 ounces of water, 3 grams of pink himalayan sea salt, and a splash of lemon juice concentrate. I sip on that for the next thirty minutes while I read and stretch. At 6 a.m., the coffee maker starts brewing my morning mud. After my coffee, I will chug another shaker bottle filled with 16 ounces of water, plus a tablespoon or more of apple cider vinegar with the "mother." So, if you do the math, I have around 45 ounces of liquids, mainly water, before 7:30 a.m. As I walk out of the door for work, I fill up an insulated water bottle with 40 more ounces of cold, filtered water that I finish before noon. At dinner, I usually sip on half of a glass of water, and then limit my fluid intake for the rest of the evening. With all of that being said, yes, I use the restroom a lot before lunch, but I'd rather need to take care of that business while I'm awake versus while I'm supposed to be asleep. Try this and see if your midnight potty breaks subside.

· · · ·

You're probably a hard worker. But unless your job requires some sort of manual labor, like construction work, plumbing, landscaping, etc., I'd venture to say that your job is more mentally taxing than truly physically taxing. Being taxed mentally can wear people down, but it won't deplete the energy systems your body has stored for physical exercise. That is why you need to exercise regularly. Of course, you want to lose fat and gain muscle from exercise, and ultimately, look good naked, but you're missing one of the greatest benefits of physical exercise: a great night's sleep! If you drain your physical energy, your body will thank you by making sure you pass out once you hit the sheets.

One thing our jobs tend to create for us is stress. If your job doesn't create stress, you still may think about it all too often, including while laying in bed at night. Once you are in bed, you shouldn't be planning out the next day's work schedule in your mind. If you have the habit of overthinking while laying in bed, it's time to find methods to make your brain be quiet. How do you accomplish this? By writing your thoughts down on paper or in a journal. Whether it's something you're stressed about, a work project, or your plan for the next day, the act of taking a pen to a piece of paper will help release those thoughts and concerns from your head.

Another great method to prevent your thoughts from racing at night is keeping and managing a calendar. At some point in the midafternoon each day, I'll take a few minutes to look at the calendar app on my phone to see what the next day holds for me. I'll add, erase, or rearrange anything that needs to be changed. This process gives me the opportunity to prioritize only my most important tasks, alleviating any feeling of being overwhelmed. This might also be helpful to you if your stress comes from procrastinating or feeling unprepared for work obligations like meetings, presentations, or projects. If simply keeping a calendar isn't relieving those anxieties, then you need to be more proactive and work on the other skills that might be causing your stress: time management, public speaking, etc. Focusing on personal development and decreasing the stressors and media in your life will be discussed later on in this book, and I feel those may help you in this situation, as well.

. . . . .

An unacceptable routine before bed involves stimulating your body and mind instead of calming them down. The main culprits of this stimulation are the electronics you are playing with and the atmosphere of the room you hang out in before going to bed, or maybe even your bedroom itself.

Each night, my wife and I make sure to turn the brightest light in our open concept living area off after we eat dinner with our daughter. Once our daughter goes to bed around 7:30 p.m., we turn the rest of the kitchen lights off, which leaves only one dimly lit lamp in the corner of the living room. At this point, we will do one last social media check for the day before we decide on what to watch for the next forty five minutes, usually a live streamed show or documentary since we've cut the cable. When the show starts, the last light is turned off, and we lay on our couch together. Yes, the TV emits stimulating light, and we have changed the brightness setting to dark in an attempt to reduce some of that, but for us, watching a show is how we decompress from our nightly playtime with our daughter and the rest of the day's events. It also allows us to connect with one another, which supports another pillar that will be discussed later in the book. But what is key for me is that once our show ends, the TV goes off, and I dive into one of my books for a minimum of twenty minutes. This is my final and most relaxing activity of the day due to its low stimulating nature.

Perhaps the biggest culprit to blame for being stimulated right before bedtime is your phone. Your phone screen emits blue light, which can reach all the way to your retina and suppress the release of melatonin, making it harder to fall asleep. The easiest way to prevent this is to turn your phone off after 7 p.m.

Now, raise your hand if you're willing to do that.

That's what I thought.

Settle down, Diane. Don't have a heart attack; there is another way. The next strategy would be to change some settings on your phone. For iPhones, there is a setting called "Night Shift," and it can be found under the display and brightness settings. I have set my phone to enter night shift from 6 p.m. to 7 a.m. daily. This setting creates an orange tint over the screen, dimming the harsh light that it usually emits. Is it perfect? No, but it's something. Beyond this quick fix, however, the ultimate goal in regard to your phone is to limit your screen time altogether (more to come on this in a later chapter).

Let's wrap this up by stating the obvious, but not so obvious strategy for better sleep: you essentially need to sleep in a cave. Your bedroom should be as dark as you can get it. You should not go to sleep with a TV on, or even better, there should not be a TV in your bedroom at all; put it elsewhere. Your bedroom should be the coziest room in your house. You should cover anything that emits light inside of your bedroom, such as an alarm clock or your phone. Preferably, you could just turn your phone off. Yes, that may require you to go buy a real alarm clock with a battery backup, just in case the electric goes out one night. If you wear a watch to track your sleep, don't let it push phone notifications to your wrist by vibrating or beeping. Your bedroom is a sanctuary. You should preserve its atmosphere at all costs. Do not do work in your bedroom. Do not watch TV in your bedroom. Do not use your phone in your bedroom. Do not argue in your bedroom. Do not have catch up conversations with your significant other in your bedroom. Do not make serious life decisions in your bedroom. The only two activities you should be doing in your bedroom are having sex and sleeping. End of story.

Chapter Notes

Three Big Takeaways

1.

2.

3.

What are your current pre and post sleep routines?

Do you currently view this pillar as a strength or a weakness?

What would you like to accomplish in regard to this pillar over the next 90 days?

12 months?

Are you committed? Can you do this?
P.S. The answer is, "Yes."

6 | PERSONAL DEVELOPMENT

It's 2019. If you are not taking opportunities to engage in personal development, then you are just making excuses. My good friend Wikipedia defines personal development as *"activities that improve awareness and identity, develop talents and potential, build human capital and facilitate employability, enhance the quality of life and contribute to the realization of dreams and aspirations."* To me, personal development is when you actively attempt to improve your life by expanding upon your skills, experience, and knowledge. There are numerous ways to accomplish this, but at the end of the day, I don't care what strategies you use, as long as you're involved in it.

"But Shawn, I can't prioritize personal development because (insert list of excuses here)." Nope. Not a reason to ignore improving yourself. Why?

BECAUSE IT'S FREE. Listening to podcasts is FREE. Signing up for email lists that send daily or weekly information tailored to your personal interests is FREE. Books are FREE. (Libraries are still a real place where you can go and check out a book, by the way!) Some seminars, both in person and online, are FREE. With the exception of hiring a real person to mentor you, all of the main avenues to develop yourself can be accessed for FREE.

But, maybe that's the problem. When something is free, it's easy to opt out. It's similar to that $10/month gym membership you've been paying for and not using. For most people, $10 isn't enough for them to get off of their couches. But did you know that your local globo gym might spend over $150 to acquire you as a new customer? Why? Because they know the average customer will spend $10/month for about three years ($360 in total + any annual "maintenance fees") before canceling a membership. That's a pretty solid return on investment. So, people are more willing to essentially throw their money away than to follow through with utilizing accessible means of self improvement.

Makes. No. Sense.

However, finding the right books, podcasts, seminars, and/or mentors is another beast entirely. They will be different for everybody.[4] It doesn't matter what your social or financial lot in life is, personal development will give you the means to further improve both.

---

[4] A few of my favorite authors and podcasters are listed in the Acknowledgement chapter.

Additionally, I would recommend studying some ideas with which you disagree. Listening to people with ideas that oppose your own is highly beneficial to understanding how others think and why they think the way they do. It allows you to ponder your own beliefs, while at the same time expand your knowledge on a topic. If you're Christian, read a book on Buddhism.[5] If you're an ultra-marathon runner, watch a few videos on strength training, or go have coffee with a local strength coach. Finding the yin to your yang and respecting the harmonious connections between the two has been lost in our society.

Don't know where to start? Read for at least fifteen minutes a day, preferably without distraction. No TV. No phone. I know others suggest reading a certain number of pages per day, but I don't want you to always stop at that number or feel forced to rush through ten pages if something on the first page makes you stop and think deeply about your current beliefs or actions.

Personally, I like to read something motivational early in the morning. I usually start reading within ten minutes of waking up. Topics that I find motivating are leadership, business, personal development, stoicism,

---

[5] I highly recommend *The Book of Joy: Lasting Happiness in a Changing World* by His Holiness the Dalai Lama and Archbishop Desmond Tutu with Douglas Abrams.

philosophy, psychology, and sociology. Two of my favorite authors are Ryan Holiday and Jim Collins. These topics and authors set my mind up to attack the day. They also make me question the beliefs, thoughts, and actions that I take with me throughout the day, and can be implemented immediately in interactions with my wife, team, or clients. My brain starts firing while reading these types of books, and as discussed in the sleep chapter, I don't want to stimulate my mind before bed, so first thing in the morning is the perfect time!

At night, I focus more on reading about historical events or biographies. I usually end up learning a lot from these books, as well, but there's a reason why I used to fall asleep in my high school history classes. It feels more like standard education than personal development. It's not boring. It's just not stimulating in the same sense as the other genres I read in the morning.

Another easy option is to listen to podcasts on the way to work or over your lunch break. You'll be amazed at the amount of information you can receive in less than a two minute drive if you have a podcast running. People make short trips all the time: to the grocery store, to the gym, to pick the kids up from school. Just because those commutes are short doesn't mean they have to be wasted time in your day. Just recently, I listened to a podcast on the way to my in-laws' house, and within the final twenty seconds of my drive, I heard two impactful statements that have resonated with me since. That moment reinforced the idea that "finding time" cannot be an excuse for not improving this particular pillar, just as it cannot be used for the others.

Another option for free personal development is to request access to private Facebook groups related to your career or a hobby, and become an active responder in those groups. Adding your thoughts to posts, and even creating posts for discussion yourself will allow you to verbalize and receive feedback on your ideas, which in turn will help broaden your knowledge and understanding of the topic.

You may be able to find a mentor for hire in one of these groups, as well. The most positive aspect of investing in a personal mentor is that he/she gets to know you and your specific situation with zero conflict of interest included. A mentor can keep an unbiased and unemotional opinion toward what your goals are and what's holding you back from reaching them. The right mentor has been through it before and has the benefit of being a Monday morning quarterback. The right mentor will also call you on your bullshit. Hindsight is 20/20, so allow him/her to be your guide into the future.

If you cannot find a mentor in your field or the investment is too high for you financially, another option is to see if your health insurance covers therapy sessions. I'm proud to say that my wife and I have been seeing a therapist for over a year, and honestly, I wish I would have started seeing one when I was a child. It feels great to talk with and listen to an unbiased professional. If you can let go of your ego, and get excited for the opportunity to improve yourself, getting called on your crap is actually an amazing feeling. Or maybe I'm just weird like that.

. . . . .

If the company you work for invests in professional development for you, I applaud them. Even though professional development helps you in regard to your career, it's ultimately done to improve the company's bottom line, not yours. An employee who advances his/her knowledge in a company's field of business, advances the company. I fully support this idea. However, an engineer who goes to a technology conference and gets to attend a small dinner with a few of the presenters may not be doing anything on the side to become a better spouse. Professional development will make you better in your career field, but not necessarily better in your life. Personal development, on the other hand, should make you better not only in your career, but every other aspect of your life, as well! Now, that's a win/win.

. . . . .

When I was a teacher, an aspect of the profession that I thoroughly enjoyed was the opportunity to learn from my own classroom lessons, figure out when something needed to be changed, and see how those changes did or did not improve them. The negative side effect of this was that when something worked, it was very easy to use it time after time without ever questioning its credibility again. After a few years of this, I became so set in my ways that I would scoff at the thought of using the newest educational tool showcased at the annual teachers summit. If it ain't broke, don't fix it, right? This is where I dropped the ball as an educator. I stopped relentlessly pursuing better strategies in the classroom. In hindsight, if I would have been involved in personal development outside of the classroom, I would have seen that improving myself on a personal level would have also benefited me on a professional level, and in turn, I would have brought that same mindset into the classroom. At that time of my life, I wasn't actively reading or listening to anything that was pulling me forward. If you find yourself in the same position, don't put your career development first. Put your personal development first, and your career will reap the benefits, as well. Don't put yourself on the back burner for the sake of making progress in only one aspect of your life.

I'm sure there are people reading this book who are so consumed by their careers that their personal relationships and health have faltered. But if I'm going to use statistics, it's also likely that over half of you aren't even engaged at work. According to a 2015 Gallup Poll, about 68% of employees are disengaged at work. So, it's safe to say that seven out of ten people who are reading this book go to work for about eight hours a day and just go through the motions until it's time to punch the clock again. Good Lord. What are you even doing with your life then? First of all, if you're disengaged at work, that is not your asshole boss's fault. It is yours. You've chosen to 1) disengage, and 2) stay at your current job. That is 100% your fault. You can choose to be engaged at work whether you're happy about your career/job or not. I've had this discussion with adults who are older than me and have a larger family than I do, and it usually ends up coming down to, "I can't just leave my job. I have a mortgage and kids to take care of." My response to those people is usually, "Well, I'm not telling you to leave your job today. But are you even actively looking for a better opportunity? Are you submitting resumes and going to interviews?" I'll let you guess what the answers to those questions usually are.

People are disengaged at work. People hate their jobs. But at the same time, PEOPLE AREN'T EVEN LOOKING FOR BETTER OPPORTUNITIES! These feelings and actions are in your control, so control them. I loved being a teacher. Were there things I didn't enjoy about being an educator? Sure. No one likes faculty meetings and hall duty and filling out paperwork that never gets looked at. But every single job, even your dream job, will have aspects that you don't enjoy. That is no reason to disengage from work and stop pursuing betterment. It is your responsibility to take ownership of the responsibilities you have as an employee. If the leadership at your company is more dictatorial than anything else, then it's on you to lead yourself. This is where personal development comes into play.

· · · · ·

Maybe you're reading this, and you've been on the reading and podcast train for a while. Awesome! If you are also involved in professional development at work, honing your skills to further your career, that's even better. You and your significant other may also be seeing a therapist, or you have stellar communication and your relationship is progressing in the right direction. I love it! So, does that mean you don't have any area of your life in which you can improve? Of course that's a rhetorical question. I hope by now you realize that you can always improve something in your life.

One thing I realized while writing this book was that I hadn't really learned anything new for myself outside of my relationship, my business, and my mindset over the past few years. Heck, to take it a step farther, I've worn gym shorts or sweats every day for the last four years. So, I started doing two new things.

First, after my morning workout, I go home, shower, and actually put real clothes on before going back to the gym to catch up on emails, or to a local coffee shop to work on other administrative tasks. You won't believe how much more productive I've become just by wearing jeans, nicer shoes, and a t-shirt that is not affiliated with my gym. If you haven't tried this life hack, I suggest you do it. I posted it to Instagram one time and I couldn't believe how many people messaged me over the next few weeks, telling me how much putting "real clothes" on improved their mood and productivity.

Secondly, I needed to find a skill to pursue that would put me back at a "beginner" level. (You know, since writing my first book isn't big enough!) I decided that, because my wife and I are taking a week long trip to Rome later this year, (our first real vacation in over three years) I would try to learn Italian. A quick post on Facebook asking friends for the best resource for learning a new language led me to an app called Duolingo. The app allows you to set the amount of time you want to dedicate to learning a new language per day. I set mine to a minimum of ten minutes. If you want to see some fun stuff, watch me use the app. I haven't tried to learn a new language since high school, over thirteen years ago. I use Duolingo every single morning before work and it makes me feel like I've accomplished something for the day before I even leave the house. The art of learning something completely new inspires productivity in a multitude of other areas. It's been a fun experience so far, learning something completely new to me. I cannot wait to show off my new language skills in front of my wife while in Rome.

Another app I recently came across and purchased was MasterClass. MasterClass "*offers online classes created for students of all skill levels*" where you can "*learn the skills essential to pursue your passion,*" or in my case, a brand new subject matter. The all-access pass cost me $180 at the time of this writing; $180 and I can watch unlimited videos from some of the world's top experts in business, writing, film, sports, music, photography, and more. The fifteen video series on writing by Malcolm Gladwell was very inspiring as I worked my way through this book. My wife has used the app to improve her photography skills. It was also pretty fun to watch the video series by Howard Schultz, the former CEO and board member of Starbucks, as I was sitting in a Starbucks, drinking a Starbucks black tea.[6]

You could also choose to learn a new task that incorporates a few of the other pillars. Sign yourself and your spouse up for dancing lessons (exercise + personal development + connection). Go on an event website, and buy a ticket to take a cooking class with a local chef (food + personal development + connection). If you and your spouse go to church but haven't done any of their events in a while, sign up for a couples discussion event (personal development + stressors / media + connection).

Anyway, if you have absolutely no clue what new skill you want to learn, close your eyes and throw a dart at the internet board. Or rediscover that hobby you abandoned as a kid or young professional. Pick something and stick with it for at least thirty days. You might be surprised how much purpose and fulfillment constantly learning brings to your life.

· · · · ·

---

[6] I'm also a huge fan of supporting your locally owned coffee shops. ;-)

In any particular area of your life, you may have one big, audacious goal, such as becoming the CEO of a company, making *The New York Times* or *Amazon* Best Sellers list, or becoming a professor at your alma mater. Whatever it is, you just can't walk around, spouting at the mouth that it's what you're going to do; you can't just wish upon a star and hope your dreams fall into your lap. You need a few secondary goals beneath that overarching one that will help elevate you to victory.

Take a look at the diagram below:

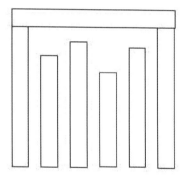

The horizontal bar, or the roof, represents the ultimate goals in your life. Everyone wants a good, solid roof over his/her head. In order to keep that roof from crumbling, the vertical bars, representing the pillars described in this book, are vital. They protect the integrity of the roof, and in turn, the entire structure. They also represent all of the minor goals you must strive toward to reach your ultimate goal. The perfect roof is one that is strongly supported by all of these pillars; there's not an Oklahoma tornado strong enough to blow that sucker off! Realistically, however, most roofs are held up by only a few vital pillars. Does that mean you can't live under that same roof? No. But is it a roof under which you want to live forever? Also, no.

We can zoom in on the shortest pillar and see that it's put together by stacking other pieces (tasks) on top of one another. In this case, let's zoom in on the fourth pillar from the left and call it the personal development pillar.

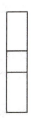

As you can see, this personal development pillar has three components. The bottom component may be fifteen minutes of reading each day. The middle component might be a short five minute video you watch over your lunch break. The top may be a few minutes of a podcast that inspires you to be a better person. In this scenario, you may time audit yourself and realize that you spent an hour or more on social media during the day, but less than an hour on developing yourself. What if you reallocated some of that mentally draining social media time to personal development? In doing so, you would add more pieces to it, eventually making it strong enough to act as another support for that metaphorical roof.

You may be thinking that all of this is fine and dandy, but how in the world are you going to add in "even more work" for yourself?! You already have a family of four, a full time job, and responsibilities to take care of at home. I don't discredit what you currently have on your plate, but from my experiences working one on one with individuals who want to take back their lives, a thorough self-audit will reveal how you are actually spending your time, and I promise you, time can be created. There are 86,400 seconds in a day. That equates to 1,440 minutes in twenty-four hours. If you just spend fifteen minutes a day on personal development, you're looking at only 1% of your day. You can't allocate 1% of your time for yourself? If you give yourself 1% a day for an entire year, in theory becoming better by 1% every day for three hundred and sixty-five days, one year from now you'll be thirty-seven times better than you are today.[7] If you're sitting here saying you don't have 1% to give to yourself, you're by default giving 99+% to someone else, correct? Who are you giving that time to? Your employer? If you work eight hours, that equals 33% of your day. Gosh, I hope you don't only live to please your boss. Are you giving that time to your family? While they are extremely important, family should be a motivation, not an excuse. After years of owning a gym, I've seen both dads and moms come in and say they've sacrificed their health to raise their children. I applaud you for your selflessness, but part of raising your children well is setting the best example possible for them. Allowing yourself to not only become stagnant, but also to regress in terms of health, wellness, and personal development is accomplishing the exact opposite. So, finding a minimum 1% of time to devote to yourself each day is not only vitally important to you, but also to your family.

. . . . .

I do not care what age you are or how long you've been stuck doing the same repeated daily tasks. You have more in you. You were made for more. You were made for better. And listen, this doesn't mean you are suddenly

---

[7] For more information, visit
https://jamesclear.com/continuous-improvement

going to take over the company you work for or somehow become an NBA all-star. I'm talking about fulfilling your life's potential, about achieving more in every aspect of your life, and doing more with the time you have left. All it takes is increasing your effort, not some innate talent that's been sitting unrecognized inside of you. America overemphasizes, even excessively sensationalizes, talent, which means we, as a collective, underemphasize everything else, including hard work and effort. It's true that working hard and giving great effort alone doesn't mean you're entitled to some high reward, a pay raise, or even praise. Working hard and putting forth an effort is just a part of doing your job, or at least that's what I believe. But sustained effort over the long term will yield huge results for you in the future, somehow, some way.

In her book *Grit: The Power of Passion and Perseverance*, Angela Duckworth, PhD, uses two equations to demonstrate the important relationship between talent and effort in terms of lifetime achievement. Her equations are based off of years of study focused on "grit" and why some people succeed, while others do not. She shows readers that if talent x effort = skill, then skill x effort = achievement.

While it's clear that your natural talent plays a role in regard to your achievement in any given activity, it is not the greatest determining factor. Dr. Duckworth states, "*Talent -- how fast we improve in skill -- absolutely matters. But effort factors into the calculations twice, not once. Effort builds skill. At the very same time, effort makes skill productive.*" In other words, just because some people have higher levels of talent at playing basketball, it doesn't mean they will ultimately excel in the sport. They may be high school standouts due to sheer size and speed, but once they get to college, where every other player has size and speed equal to (if not greater than) them, the true separator becomes effort. Anyone who has been around a college or NFL football team, or has any knowledge about the history of the sport, understands that being a college standout doesn't equate to professional achievement in the sport (Ryan Leaf anyone?).

Why does this matter to you? Chances are you're not trying to enter the NBA draft next year, and you're just wondering what to make your family of four for dinner tonight. Perfect. You probably aren't trying to become the best in the world at something, but it's likely that you have become content with being average or stagnant in terms of the goals you once pursued passionately. I'm here to tell you, that's not good enough. If you feel like you've tapped out on your skill level, I need you to realize that putting a little more effort into your work or a particular task will not only increase your skills at said task, but according to Dr. Duckworth's research, it will increase your achievement in relation to that skill, or in this case, your life.

Maybe you don't think you have any talent. Maybe you think every skill you have is a fixed trait and you can't improve. Maybe you're afraid of failure. Maybe you're not sure what life could look like if you pursued more for yourself. I can't pinpoint what it is that causes your hesitation, but I do know this: fear, whether it's the fear of failure, fear of judgement, or even fear of success, is a self-fulfilling prophecy. Remember, you must relentlessly pursue a better you. You're not trying to earn a spot on some "Sleep All-Star Team" or the "USA Olympic Team of Personal Development." You're not being put up against everyone else or the best in the world. You are making yourself better. You are here to take back your life and continuously move forward from now until the day you die.

· · · · ·

My hope is that this chapter has motivated you to take action, but I want to reiterate that I'm not here to motivate you. Motivation is fleeting. It's a short-term fuel for something that is a long-term journey. When you start reading and listening to podcasts, the ideas you glean from those sources will help you identify all kinds of things you could be doing better, and they will resonate with you. But I promise you, acknowledgement alone will not give you the drive to entirely change your behavior. That doesn't mean you're a hopeless failure. Embrace the challenge of in-the-moment self-awareness rather than fearing it or judging yourself because of it.

Your thoughts, just like your physical actions, have become a part of your muscle memory. It's going to take time to actually adjust your thinking and responses to situations. Last week, my wife reorganized the floating shelf above our coffee maker. The jar of coffee used to be on the far left. It's now in the middle, which is literally only four inches to the right. It's been a few days since she made this small change, but even this morning, after pouring the water into the coffee machine, I reached up without looking and accidentally grabbed the coconut oil, which is now on the far left side of the shelf. Without looking, I put it back and grabbed the next thing in line, which was the bag of cacao butter. Only after recognizing I had the cacao butter in my hand did I actually look up to find the coffee. Five days after this change, it still took me three failed attempts to realize I actually had to look to grab the correct item. This is true for any change, no matter how small, and will absolutely hold true in terms of your own personal development. Your behaviors will not change overnight, but with consistent effort, they will eventually change.

· · · · ·

When people are lacking motivation in life, many say they need to be pushed to take steps toward changing. You shouldn't look to push or be pushed. Even I'm not here to push you. Pushing requires someone else to get behind you. In other words, to drop down a level. Instead, you should look to pull and be pulled forward by someone who is where you want to be. Others shouldn't have to drop down a level to get you to lurch forward with them. You should accelerate your efforts, education, and discipline to rise up to where you want to be. As they pull you, you will learn the necessary steps to stay in a place where you desire to be. I want to pull you forward. I want you to find other people who want to pull you forward. Pull, not push.

· · · · ·

Skill development and provoking a deeper understanding of yourself, your views, and the world around you will take you from being okay to being good, from good to great, and from great to untouchable. But the process is not a "one shot and done," or an "every now and then" pursuit. It needs to be relentlessly pursued by you, for you. Personal development doesn't seek your attention. It doesn't come to you. You go to it. You undertake the responsibility to join the race. The marathon that is personal development is always moving forward. It's never-ending. The differentiator is whether or not you register for the race, and then, continue to run.

Fitting, considering I just signed up for my 1st 10K as part of USMC Marathon.

#universe

Chapter Notes

Three Big Takeaways

1.

2.

3.

What do you currently do for personal development?

Do you currently view this pillar as a strength or a weakness?

What would you like to accomplish in regard to this pillar over the next 90 days?

12 months?

Are you committed? Can you do this?
P.S. The answer is, "Yes."

7 | STRESSORS / MEDIA

Strain. Pressure. Nervous Tension. Worry. Anxiety. Trouble. Difficulty. Hassle. Those are some of the synonyms Google provides for the word "stress." Also according to Google, stress can be defined as *"a state of mental, physical, or emotional strain or tension resulting from adverse or very demanding circumstances."*

Notice that it says no where in the definition that stress is a "negative" strain or tension. Stress can be beneficial to the human body and mind, if you know how to respond to it properly. Without stress, you don't push your body to new levels when you are working out. Without stress, you aren't able to push your mind to comprehend new information or concepts. After you read this book, and you stop eating crap food, stop treating yourself like crap, and stop making ridiculous excuses for negative behaviors, your body and mind will encounter some high quality stress. Trust me. But if you learn how to work through the stress and push beyond it, so many positive things will come from that short term strain.

The stress I'm going to focus on in this chapter is the stress from events you control. The stress you get from what you willingly put in front of your own face. The stress that results from what you watch and read on any media outlet, particularly social media. The stress that you encounter in your life due to events outside of your direct control will be addressed in a future chapter. But skipping ahead would be detrimental to your forward progress. ==The fact is that you cannot properly combat stress from things outside of your control until you know how to curtail the stress within your control.==

    I've debated, and still am debating, calling this chapter "Stress Media" because most of my discussion revolves around the stress you're willingly participating in when you interact with social media. Did you catch that? You. You're the one choosing what you're viewing on social media, not the social media platform.

    The unfortunate truth is that anger and rage are the most dominant and viral emotions elicited by social media. The internet is one of, if not the, greatest inventions of all time. Social media, however, is the cancer that is causing it to rot from the inside. What's even worse, though, is that we have the ability to either feed that cancer or cure it, and boy, are we feeding it.

    I'm not saying you should delete all of your social media accounts and live the rest of your life without it. I am actually a huge fan of social media, especially Facebook and Instagram. They are primarily the means by which I share my message with the world, and an incredibly effective way for my business to get its brand out to the local community. Social media plays a positive role in my life, but that's because I've chosen to use it in a positive way.

. . . . .

Most social media platforms, especially Facebook, have touted the desire to build communities and bring people together. So how can anger and hostility be the most prominent emotions produced by engaging with it? I'm not smart enough to provide a perfectly scientific answer (actually I will take a shot… it's because people are frustrated with themselves because they don't exercise, don't eat right, don't sleep well, don't do anything positive to develop their abilities, don't know how to handle stress properly, and don't connect with the right people in the right way… sounds like the foundations of a damn good book if you ask me!), but I have a few strategies that will prevent you from continuing to feed this disease.

I'm about to give you possibly the most beneficial piece of advice contained within this book. It's easier than exercise. It's easier than eating healthy food. It's just as refreshing as sleep. It will be one huge step toward increasing your personal development, and it will help you create better connections in your life (something I'll address in the next chapter). Are you ready for this?

==I'm giving you permission to unfollow and unfriend whoever the fuck you want on social media without justification.==

Extra space for emphasis.

Another extra space for double emphasis.

Go back up and read it again.

You know how we do it.

A little louder for the people in the back.

You have zero control of most of the things that happen around you on a daily basis. ==But what you read, what you see, what you engage in, and who you follow on social media is 100% within your control.== So start taking control of it, Karen!

I guarantee you are already thinking of someone on your newsfeed who gets on your nerves every time he/she posts something. For most of you, it might be that one person who can't even find something positive in a slow motion video of golden retriever puppies running across a freshly mowed back yard. You know, the person who has a problem for every solution.

Do you have that person in mind?

Okay. Stop reading, pull out your phone, go to each of your social media accounts, and unfollow or unfriend that person right now. If you never interact with that person, unfriending is a good option. If you're worried about any kickback from unfriending that person (you shouldn't be, but I understand if you are) just unfollow him/her. Facebook provides no indication that you have unfollowed someone, so that person will remain none the wiser that you've made any changes.

Do it right now.

Right now.

Do not move on in this book until you do this one simple, yet vitally important, task. Everyone reading this book can find ==at least one person who is pushing him/her backward instead of pulling him/her forward.==

Wow. How did that feel?!

Freaking refreshing, right?!

It was also empowering, wasn't it? And not in an "I'm better than you" kind of way. More so in an "I can do this. I have control over what I want to see on MY social media" kind of way. Congratulations! You just took one step toward de-stressing your life.

Your health doesn't just involve your body's physical state. It includes your mind, as well, and this step will move you in the right direction. You wouldn't allow someone to come up and punch you every single day, so why are you voluntarily handing over your thoughts and feelings to others by allowing their social media posts to frustrate you? This isn't referring to you posting your thoughts and feelings. This is referring to you allowing those on social media to negatively influence your mind. You may not even realize how much you're doing this, but it is self-inflicted. You must start protecting your sanity through regulating what you're seeing and who you're seeing it from. Stop scrolling through someone else's social media life and start living your real life.

· · · · ·

In the words of the great Roman emperor, Marcus Aurelius, "*It never ceases to amaze me: we all love ourselves more than other people, but care more about their opinions than our own.*" It is true that social media has empowered every single person to use his/her voice, but look at the way you use your social media. You read more about other people's opinions than you post about your own. You end up allowing others' opinions to influence how you think and feel about the decisions you have made. Here is a tactic that I have found beneficial throughout my use of social media: when I post something about my life and someone counters it with his/her opinion, I politely respond that I am not looking for opinions, only to share my experience. My posts are never meant to force my thoughts onto other people, nor to expose myself to people who disagree with me. While there are times when I'm open to disagreement, I get to decide when I'm looking or asking for someone else's opinion. It's okay to let people know when they can keep their thoughts to themselves. This is how you'll protect your sanity if/when you choose to use social media.

  Marcus Aurelius is also known for saying, "*We have the power to hold no opinion about a thing and to not let it upset our state of mind--for things have no natural power to shape our judgements.*" Imagine that. These ideas are coming from someone who was writing his personal philosophies between the years 161-180 AD, long before the internet and social media existed. Think about all of the things you read online that make you roll your eyes in frustration. How many of them are you thoroughly knowledgeable about? Yet, how many of them do you respond to, only to end up in a silly argument that took up way too much of your personal time? It's okay to have no opinion whatsoever about a particular person or situation. But for some reason, we care so much about addressing those outside factors that we are willing to compromise our own emotional and mental wellbeing to do so. Ignorance can be bliss, but not giving a shit about 99% of the things you see on the internet, or even most of the things happening around you, will protect your sanity.[8]

. . . . .

Unfollowing and unfriending the high level complainers is the easy part. What will take more time and effort is actually unfollowing the people who you think are there to motivate, inspire, and pull you forward, but are actually making you feel inferior.

During the first few years of using CrossFit as my main source of exercise, I wanted to see how far I could go in "the sport of fitness." I was pushing my body to the extremes. I'd work out early in the morning, go to work, and then get right back to the gym. So, of course, I started following the highest level athletes in the sport on social

---

[8] For more on Stoic Philosophy, I recommend reading Ryan Holiday and Stephen Hanselman's *The Daily Stoic*.

media. I wanted to be like them. They inspired me. They motivated me. I was learning from the videos they shared.

Fast forward a few years, when I made the decision to take a step back from such high level training in order to focus on my spouse and business. I reduced my training time from three hours per day to a single, one hour class. My goal changed from wanting to be competitive to just wanting to be healthy, uninjured, and happy with devoting more time to my family and business. But I kept following the high level athletes on social media.

It took me awhile, but one day I realized that seeing videos of them working out and competing wasn't bringing me joy anymore. Seeing pictures of guys hitting new personal records on their lifts made me think, "Ah man, I'm nowhere near that strong anymore." I began feeling inferior to people who had completely different goals than me. They weren't posting anything negative, but the way I was interpreting what I was seeing was making me doubt what I was doing. So, one by one, I unfollowed all of them.

Maybe you aren't trying to compete in a sport or follow high level athletes, but you are interested in fashion and makeup, so you follow a few of the top bloggers in that space on social media. There's no problem with that. But let's say you're a forty-five year old mother who has a full time job, and you just want to learn some new techniques to apply your makeup, or what colors should be in your wardrobe this season. Let's also say you follow a twenty-five year old "blogger" who, whether you know it or not, lives at home off of an inheritance and has a friend who does video editing and photoshopping for free. Her friend makes her look flawless in every single photo she posts. Even though you learn something from her here or there, ultimately, you are comparing yourself to her. But you're not twenty-five anymore, and looking at her posts only makes you feel bad about yourself. It's time to take the power back and click that unfollow button.

Question everything and everyone you follow. Are they adding real value to your life? Is stopping your thumb scroll to see their pictures and read their captions truly making you happy? If the answer is no, cut them out of your feed. Or, as Marie Kondo would say, thank them for their time in your life, but they no longer bring you joy, and throw them away.

・ ・ ・ ・ ・

Take control of the algorithm of your life. The way Facebook's algorithm works is based on the things you "like." The algorithm uses that information to push similar content your way. It is creating a digital menu of what you like, and feeding it to you even when you aren't hungry. Certain people view this as a problem. I don't. The real problem is that you are "liking" things you don't actually like. For example, say your best friend goes on a negative Nancy rant about the President and this policy or that policy. You, on the other hand, don't really care about politics, but just because she is your friend, you "like" her status. Well, you just told the algorithm that you like when people rant about politics. Keep it coming, Facebook!

  A professional acquaintance of mine recently posted the following as her Facebook status: "*Ah, Facebook. I don't know if I can take the heartache anymore of the low vibe newsfeed. So much anger, judgment, hostility, blame, and on, and on, and on. What you think about, you bring about. Speak what you seek until you see what you said. Gratitude, compassion, understanding, peacefulness, wisdom, love. I'm gonna hang out with my kids, read some books, do some yoga, hug some trees, meditate, and find some ways to spread kindness. If you wanna chat, text or call me. Taking a temporary hiatus.*" The comments ranged anywhere from "*It's the way of the elite. Turn us all against each other to ensure control. Divide and conquer*" to "*Facebook is so depressing right now in a lot of ways.*" I simply replied with, "Then start unfollowing and unfriending people. You control your feed by who you associate with on the platform." If you're that caught up in the negative atmosphere you're seeing on social media, going cold turkey and ditching it altogether might be a good idea, but if we are being real with each other, you will be back on the platform in thirty days. You probably aren't going to just give up on Facebook or Instagram, where you have hundreds of pictures of your kids and the best times of your life stored. So, the better option is to start controlling the data going into the algorithm. Luckily, this friend of mine took my advice and posted the following day that she will "*start choosing who I want in my feed. But I am not going to stay off of Facebook and miss the friends and business page posts that contribute to my happiness, laughter, and high vibe increase.*" Yes! That's what it's about: you taking control of what you see!

. . . . .

Now, let's move on to a whole other beast of a stressor.

Your phone.

It's right next to you, isn't it? You can see it or feel it from where you're sitting.

I want you to do something. Close your eyes and imagine your phone is in an entirely different room than where you are currently sitting. Solely focus on that scenario for thirty seconds, and note how your body and mind react.

I created this little activity for a seminar I was hosting a few months ago, and when I did it myself, I got really uncomfortable. Even though my eyes were closed, I felt them wanting to look in the direction of the room I was imagining[9]. This may sound weird, but I literally felt my heart being pulled toward my phone. Did you get anxious and imagine yourself getting up to retrieve it? I did. Maybe I'm the only person who felt that way during this exercise, but I'm going to venture to say that I'm not. In fact, I'd even wager a bet that the majority of you don't quite remember the last time you intentionally chose to disengage from your phone, to turn it off, or leave it in another room for a prolonged period of time (an hour, or even more).

Want to know how I got this book typed up? By turning my phone off for one full hour every day from Monday through Friday until it was done. It's the only way this book could have come to fruition. Not only did I finish this book, but another amazing thing happened (or, rather,

---

[9] My phone was actually in another room, so I wasn't really imagining this. If you are imagining this and don't feel anything, go put your phone in another room and try again.

didn't happen) while my phone was off. I did not miss a single emergency. My business did not go bankrupt or collapse. My wife didn't obsessively try to text or call me, then get mad at me for not answering. My world did not fall apart during the months it took to write this book. Despite my anxiety at even the thought of leaving my phone in another room when I started this process, being without it for sixty minutes each day proved to be inconsequential.

When I'm trying to make a point, I like to remove all of the fluff around the situation or object, so let's do that with your phone. You are dependent on that little, square piece of technology that's currently sitting on the coffee table next to you or in your pocket. It is created out of nothing more than plastic, metal, and wires. And yet, it has so much power over you that even imagining that it was outside of your immediate reach caused a physical response of anxiety. That's dependency. Sound familiar? It should. It's the same response alcoholics have when they run out of booze, or the feeling drug addicts have when they don't have a hit.

· · · · ·

I'm not naive, though. We need our phones. We need them for emergencies. We need them for communication. We need them for work. We need them to be productive. We need them to save time. We need them to quickly order more copies of this book for our best friends while we are thinking about it.

    My phone, even though it is off, is sitting a thumb's length away from the side of my laptop as I type this sentence. Yes, I stopped typing and measured the distance with my thumb. I did not leave it in my car because, you know, someone could walk by, break my window, search every little crevice of my vehicle, find my phone under my seat, and steal it… duh, that could definitely happen, so why would I EVER leave my phone in my car?![10] You need your phone, but you don't really NEED your phone attached to your hip at all times, nor do you need to immediately stare at it whenever you have a break in the day or are bored. But you've become addicted to your phone, and now your brain aches for that little bit of dopamine that you get whenever you lift your phone up and see that little, red notification symbol. And you are the person who trained it to do that.

    Apps are created to do one thing: keep you on them. The colors, the gamification, and yes, the pop up alerts

---

[10] With my luck, half of the people reading this book are included in the small percentage whose phones have actually been stolen from their cars.

letting you know when someone liked something of yours, were all created to keep you coming back for more of that candy. You unlock your phone and see a red circle with a number five in it pop up from the Instagram app. Drip. Dopamine is released into your brain. Someone commented on your #fitness photo from earlier today! Drip. And, burmp, it was a robot who is set to auto-comment. "Hey you! Much like pic! We look for brand ambassadors just like you. Follow us asap!" Womp. Womp. Womp. What a let down. But, hey, at least your brain got the good ole drip drip.

This is when you need to sell yourself on the idea that the world inside of your phone is not as important as the world outside of it. Turn off all the notifications from as many apps as you can. No push notifications. No banner alerts. No little red circles. None of them. Take similar apps and put them in their own folders instead of allowing them to stand alone on the screen. Finally, remove all of those apps and folders from your home screen. Move everything to the second and third screen on your phone. Now your home screen will be a beautiful picture of your family, or a quote that reminds you to relentlessly pursue a better you (you can find a few of these quotes on Instagram @therelentlesspursuitofyou).

When you're out with friends and family, or working on important tasks, put your phone face down. ==When you take your significant other out for dinner, only take one phone, and seriously consider leaving it in the car.== It's extremely sad to my wife and I when we go out to dinner and notice how many people are on their phones while waiting for their food. The worst I've seen is a family of six, including a mom, dad, three kids, and a grandparent, out to dinner at a nice restaurant, all with their eyes glued to their phone screens. When you are in the presence of someone you care for, who is special to you, give that person your attention. Connect with him/her, not what's on your phone.

· · · · ·

All of the suggestions provided in this chapter are simple, but not easy. Most of the information in this book has encouraged you to actively and consistently make positive choices to benefit your body and mind. But this chapter is pretty much just asking you to "set it and forget it." It is really simple to change your notification settings and move the apps around on your screen, but the black hole that is social media has an unrelenting pursuit of its own. It sucks us back in from time to time. If you heed the warnings of phone addiction, you'll reap the benefits of being more present in what matters most: your real life and the real people around you, who not only vie for your attention, but deserve it.

Chapter Notes

Three Big Takeaways

1.

2.

3.

What do you currently do for stressors / media?

Do you currently view this pillar as a strength or a weakness?

What would you like to accomplish in regard to this pillar over the next 90 days?

12 months?

Are you committed? Can you do this?
P.S. The answer is, "Yes."

8 | CONNECTION

    Let's imagine we are juggling a few balls in the air. One ball is your career, another is your relationship, and the last is your personal health and development, all of which are vitally important. But, what you don't realize is that the latter two are made of glass. If you drop them, they hit the ground and break into a million pieces. Can you glue them back together so they are exactly the same as they once were? Sure. But, that takes a while. It would have been a lot easier to keep those two balls in the air in the first place. However, the unscathed ball, representing your career, is made of rubber. If you drop it, it will always bounce back. There will always be opportunities for jobs, as long as you are ready to catch them when they come in your direction. The glass balls, therefore, should be kept in the air at all costs.

    But if you are looking at your feet right now and have no place to step where a shard won't stab you in the foot because you simultaneously dropped your health and relationship balls, you have to acknowledge that. You can't just remain standing in the same place for the rest of your life. Let's get down and start picking up the pieces.

Realistically, I'm not writing this chapter for you. I'm writing it for me. Building strong, growing relationships has been one of my biggest weaknesses throughout life. Improving this pillar has only recently become a focus of mine. There have been so many reasons for me to avoid this in the past. As a young man, I was too shy to put myself out there enough to build relationships. In both high school and college, I used football as my excuse; I didn't want a girlfriend to distract me from achieving my athletic goals. As college came to a close, I decided I wanted to eventually move closer to my childhood home in Pennsylvania, so I didn't want to get "too close" with anyone in North Carolina. I've had close friends throughout my life, but when we weren't together, or eventually lived farther apart, I did nothing to continue cultivating and growing those relationships. Call it silly, but that's how my brain worked.

I'm an introvert, and even though I enjoy public speaking, I don't get energized by being around huge crowds, or people, in general. I am energetic when I'm on stage, but once I'm done "entertaining," I just want to go lay down.

"We are social beings." "We need other people." "We need deeply connected relationships to survive." I've heard these phrases stated as fact in a variety of circumstances throughout my life, but I never believed them. Here I was, an introvert who didn't like talking to strangers, and I didn't really understand that those commonly used statements didn't actually mean I needed to talk to people all of the time. They just mean that I need to be close to a select handful of people who I can really, truly get to know.

    For most of my life, being a part of a team that required the efforts of a group of people to be successful was how I cultivated relationships and made connections with others. In school, I wasn't the class clown, and I hardly ever rose my hand to answer questions, even if I knew the answer, because I didn't want to talk. But on the football field, all I had to do was execute my responsibilities. The team's collective actions did all of the communicating. In this sense, I wasn't required to talk, just to block, tackle, score touchdowns, and let the scoreboard speak for me. If you were in the same boat as I was, you eventually realized that this type of expression just wouldn't cut it, especially in the workplace. This became apparent to me when I decided to become a high school teacher and start a gym.

· · · · ·

Years later, I have finally admitted to myself that my lack of deep connections wasn't a result of my introverted nature; it was because I was extremely selfish. I wanted to succeed in football so I could get a scholarship to college, earn the recognition that came along with it, and eventually become a highly touted college athlete. In my eyes, any person who wanted to spend time with me soon became a hindrance who needed to be shut out. I had a big, audacious goal, and if you couldn't directly help me reach it, I turned a blind eye to your needs.

The last semester of high school, when students should be having the time of their lives with their best friends, became a time when I started to shut out all of the friends I had played football with for the previous eight years. I started hanging out with a few "new" friends because, deep down, I felt it would be easier to cut them off once I left for college. At this point, every single one of my friends had decided to go to in-state universities. However, I had chosen a school located eight hours and four states away, where I knew no one, and where I also knew that no one from my hometown, besides my family, would come visit me. During my four years of college, only two of my friends from high school came to visit me on a single occasion. And honestly, that was entirely okay with me, a reflection of my inability and lack of desire to cultivate relationships.

As I sit here and write this out, I'm actually starting to feel sad about the way I subconsciously made all of these decisions. It's crazy to think back and realize that I was pushing people away without even knowing why, yet now it's so clear to me. My connection pillar was most certainly the weakest one of them all because I avoided deep, meaningful relationships at all costs. But thankfully, I have been building it up slowly over the past few years.

. . . . .

I met my wife at 5:45 one morning when she walked into our gym. She had lost a push-up contest to a friend over the weekend, and her "punishment" was to come with him to a CrossFit class the following Monday morning. She was the antithesis of who I was at the time: bubbly, talkative, and constantly smiling.

She put up with a lot of superficial, unfulfilling communication during those first few years of our relationship. Growing the gym had my full attention, just as football had in my past. I'm surprised she stuck with me; I would find any excuse to be at the gym "in order for it to stay afloat." This may have been another attempt to avoid getting too close to someone, for me to stay selfish and focus only on something bigger than myself. But deep down, I knew she was what and who I needed. She was my missing puzzle piece. The ying to my yang. The peanut butter to my jelly. The mayonnaise to my pancake. Oh wait… sick of me yet? Honestly, she was the whole damn pillar that I was missing.

Fast forward a few years, and we are married with two energetic goldendoodles and a beautiful baby girl. I've learned a few things about connection throughout that time, but I am far from where I'd like to be. It's a constant work in progress to let go of my ego and put as much effort into improving relationships as I do with myself. I do believe you need to put yourself first, but the gap I placed between myself and others was vast. That gap is narrowing daily.

· · · · ·

Once I realized I didn't need to be an extrovert and talk to every person on the planet to have deep, meaningful connections, I was able to slowly open the door to let some people get to know me and vice versa. Owning a micro gym was the perfect scenario for me. I could interact with a group of people for an hour at a time. I could slowly learn about the lives of the people in my classes without feeling forced or overwhelmed.

As our gym grew, I learned about a theory known as Dunbar's Number, a *"suggested cognitive limit to the number of people with whom one can maintain stable social relationships."* British anthropologist, Robin Dunbar, believes that most people can only have stable relationships with one hundred and fifty people until the quality of those relationships start to deteriorate. In the micro gym industry, Dunbar's Number holds true; if the staff to client ratio requires each employee to maintain more than one hundred and fifty relationships, the quality of gym instruction and client satisfaction begins to falter. The first time our gym hit two hundred members, we went right back down to one hundred and fifty over the course of the next three months because it was the first time we had to service and cultivate relationships with that many people. We were not ready to handle the workload, and because we could not build and sustain that many relationships, people cancelled their memberships. It was a beneficial personal and professional learning experience about the "more isn't always better" mentality. Better is better. Building quality, sustainable relationships with a smaller amount of people will have a more profound impact on your life than attempting to acquire a long list of people who remain simple acquaintances.

For me, having less than five extremely close friends has been a good start to laying a solid foundation for my connection pillar. I obviously associate with more people than that, but rarely beyond simple pleasantries (deep conversation is still a struggle for me). When I am talking about true connections, I mean people with whom I can share my honest and controversial opinions, rely on to offer sound advice, etc. I can think of no more than five people who fit that description.

It's commonly said that your income is relatively close to the average income of the five people you associate with on a regular basis. So, in other words, if you add together the income of the five people you see the most and divide the total by five, that number will be close to your personal income. I'm going to add a few more layers to this principle. The five people who are the closest with you likely also share similar attitudes, desires, work ethics, mindsets, levels of ambition, and disciplined habits. Do you have a friend who is constantly complaining? That rubs off on you. Do you have another friend who blames his/her spouse for everything going wrong in life? That rubs off on you, too. Does one (or more) of your friends avoid the gym and invite you to come over to destroy two bottles of wine on a Tuesday night? That certainly rubs off on you. When you start to audit your life and make changes in order to

==better yourself, a byproduct of this will be leaving a few people behind.== And that's okay because it might mean that you instead spend that random Tuesday night finishing a tough workout while your friend cheers you on, or discussing the many reasons that you are still so in love with your partner. Those are the things that build solid, positive connections.

· · · · ·

The most powerful connection you can have is with a significant other, but somehow much of our society has forgotten its value, as the divorce rate in the United States alone is nearly fifty percent. I'm not here to fix the marriage problem, or to tell you that people shouldn't get divorced because, quite frankly, I look around and see a lot of couples who should get divorced. But, with that being said, I also see too many people prematurely giving up on themselves, giving up on their partners, and in turn, giving up on potentially the most important connection in their lives. Before you pull the trigger and go the divorce route, maybe you should ask yourself if you have legitimately made an effort to fix yourself, not your partner.

Just trying to be nice to your spouse for one day isn't good enough. When my wife and I went through some struggles in the past, I remember being intentional about making singular kind gestures in hopes of showing her that I was trying harder, and if it wasn't received well, I'd get all butthurt and give up for another few days. Talk about the opposite of "relentless pursuit." But that's exactly where you may be in your relationship. You've not only stopped relentlessly pursuing a better life for yourself, you've also stopped relentlessly pursuing a better relationship with the person you love... or once loved.

One day, while writing this book at a local coffee shop, a husband and wife sat down next to me. I'm a huge people watcher, and I become keenly aware of how people interact with one another in public places. They were waiting on a business acquaintance. While waiting, they hardly talked, but when they did, it was very unemotional, low toned, even defensive. At one point, the wife asked her husband if he wanted to try her coffee (I use the term coffee lightly because hers looked more like a caramel milkshake). He declined with a simple, "No." She asked again. He declined with a slightly annoyed, "No." Finally, she said, "I was just trying to see if you wanted to taste something new." He mumbled something else as he looked at his paperwork, at which point I glanced at his wife to get her reaction. She rolled her eyes, moved her coffee to her other hand, and literally turned her back to her husband. For the next ten minutes, the husband did not say a word to his wife. I'll be the first to admit that I have no clue what was going on in their lives, but that situation and what occurred next is something I feel happens all too often. As soon as their acquaintance showed up, they both came alive! They smiled at him, talked loudly, were energetic, and extremely attentive, not only to him, but to each other.

I've been there and done that, and I'm here to say that it is wrong. It's assbackwards. ==If you talk to other people with fresh enthusiasm, yet talk to your significant other as if you're annoyed, you need to fix your shit.==

After witnessing this scenario, I posted it on social media to see what other people thought about the interaction, and hopefully get them to think about how they regularly interact with their own spouses. A female member of my gym messaged me asking for any advice on how to "fix the shit" as she and her husband "have been stuck for awhile." I asked, "What car do you drive?" After she replied, my next question was, "How many of that same car do you see each day now that you've bought it?" Her answer? "About 5 or so."

Here was my response verbatim: "Right. When we view our spouses as annoying, or we bring frustrations from outside of the house to the inside, all we're going to see is annoying and frustrating behavior. Even when our spouses are doing something sweet, we'll still feel annoyed and frustrated. So, we have to be intentional at looking for the good, at taking on the responsibility of thanking them when they do something nice. The more we affirm them, the more we will see the positive in them, and in ourselves. And when they actually do something annoying, we need to ask ourselves, 'Is this really a big deal in the grand scheme of my life, or our life as a couple?'"

    Let's go back to the couple at the coffee shop. Even though that entire situation could be seen by others as insignificant, I think it is a big deal. Both spouses could have handled it better, and communicated with each other in a nicer way. It's on both of them. First of all, when asked if he wanted to try his wife's drink, the husband could have simply made eye contact, smiled, and said, "No, thank you." Or, he could have said, "Yes," and taken a very little sip of his wife's coffee, even if he only drinks black coffee. Bam. Frustrating situation averted! Or, after he said, "No," the wife could have changed the topic instead of asking him another time. She could have taken a sip, and said, "It actually tastes like that caramel dessert you like from your favorite restaurant." And if he said, "No," again, she could have made a joke: "Suit yourself; I'll just be over here having an orgasm in my mouth." Dang! That would have gotten his attention, wouldn't it have?! Sure, they could have been a nice, reserved couple that doesn't use the word orgasm in public, but geez! Can we start being playful with one another again? Oh, but it can't be that simple, right? Yes, it can be!

The point is that there are always more constructive ways to respond to our spouses, even if their behavior seems annoying in the moment. It's important to actively make the decision to respond in a positive way, rather than letting ourselves get consumed by negativity that will roll over into other parts of our relationships.

. . . . .

Although not every couple is willing to use the word "orgasm" in public as suggested in the previous scenario, it does bring me to another vital aspect of improving spousal connections: being playful! Bringing playfulness back into your relationship, just like every other thing mentioned in this book, won't happen overnight. But, if you make an effort at increasing the amount of playful banter you have with your partner, I promise you that the byproduct will be something we all desire, yet don't participate in enough with our partners: various forms of intimacy, including (insert shocked emoji here) sex!

I get it. You aren't some young horny jackrabbit any longer. You've been married for more years than you care to count, and you think that just because I'm thirty and only four years deep into marriage, I don't know what I'm talking about. You're one of those people who would tell me, "Just wait. Eventually, sex will be nonexistent." It's kind of like when I was twenty and people who were older and out of shape told me, "Just wait until you turn thirty and have a job. You'll gain weight." And now that I'm thirty, everyone who is older is telling me, "Just wait." You know what? I will wait. I will wait until I'm forty to prove them wrong. It's the same case with couples who are no longer intimate with one another. You think it's just normal to stop having sex with your spouse as you get older, are raising a family, and work demands have doubled. I'm not buying it. Did you stop having sex in college when you had three papers, four finals, and a group project due all at once? Nope.

I just think the people who believe such a thing can't admit what's actually happened. They've let themselves go. They no longer exercise. They eat like assholes, which makes them feel like crap. They don't sleep well for a multitude of reasons. They haven't learned anything or developed a skill in years. They are essentially living the same life from ten years ago. They care more about what Sally from down the street is posting about her family on Instagram than paying attention to their own families' true desires for attention. See what I'm getting at? Their connection pillars are lacking because the others are lacking, too. And it's because of all of these factors that they no longer want to be intimate with anyone.

You know what? I bet if I did all of those things, I wouldn't be having sex either. Bringing all of that negative junk into your relationship, coupled with a partner who is doing the same thing, and you have a recipe for disaster. I hope this isn't the case, but I bet all of the things I just described resonated with some people who are reading this book. If you let yourself go like this, if you stop relentlessly pursuing a better you, your desire for intimacy is going to dissipate.

And I'm not saying you need to be a Victoria's Secret model in order to feel desirable or want to be intimate because I don't think that is what makes someone sexy. Now, this is my personal opinion, but there is nothing more attractive in this world than someone who recognizes the opportunity to grow in a variety of aspects of his/her life, and then seizes those opportunities. I may be the only person in the world who thinks that, and if I am, then you can rip this section out of the book, but I bet if you thought about it, you'd find that kind of ambition sexy, too.

With that being said, if you start working on yourself, your partner isn't going to suddenly pounce on you, and it shouldn't work that way. Honestly, if you start working on yourself, especially after years of being stagnant, your partner may actually get mad and frustrated. If so, keep "doing you" emotionally, mentally, and physically (after all, an orgasm is an orgasm whether your partner gets you there or you do it yourself). Once you start seeing the positive effects of more consistent exercise, better eating and sleeping habits, personal development, and lower stress levels, your partner will notice, and either 1) want to join you in your journey, or 2) continue to be a miserable cow. Keep going. He/she may come around eventually, but it won't be instantaneous unless you embarked on this journey together. In fact, it might help to encourage your spouse to read this book, as well. However, you should avoid doing what I initially did when I started reading literature of this nature. I used the books I was reading to point out to my wife everything she was "doing wrong" when she hadn't even read the books I was referring to. The way I presented personal growth tactics to my wife was wrong. Lesson learned.

If after a while, your husband, "Too Good For Personal Growth Paul," still isn't catching on to your hints at affection and that you're pushing this train forward with or without consent, the two of you will need to decide what happens next. But, my honest belief is that both partners need to work on themselves and their relationship. It's not just on one person's plate. And if one partner isn't game for this journey and the other is… well, that's when I applaud the person who goes to the divorce attorney. Perhaps you have an entirely different view on this, and believe that no one should get a divorce. I respect your thoughts, but I'd love to hear your justification as to why someone should have to go through life with someone who puts no effort into personal improvement, and, in turn, his/her relationship. Don't worry, I'll wait.

My wife and I are real people. We disagree. We bicker. We argue. We say things we shouldn't, and respond to each other the wrong way more times than we'd like to admit. But where we are today is a lot better than where we were in the past. I remember the day when everything changed between us. We were sitting on the couch together while our daughter was taking a nap, and we admitted something extremely difficult to each other. Our relationship was not the type that either of us wanted. If we did not start working on our issues, both individually and as a couple, there was only one place where this train would stop. We looked at each other, no tears in our eyes (yet), and uttered the word "divorce" to one another. It was the first time we had ever used that word out loud, and, in the moment, we remained unemotional. We did not yet grasp the magnitude of the suggestion, but it wouldn't take long until the weight of it came crashing down on both of us.

Do you want to know what we did after that? We changed our actions toward one another. We started to work out our personal issues without judging each other for doing so. Now, we aren't perfect, but we are more understanding of each other's needs. We are more open to being called out when we are falling back into old habits. We are more prone to stop in the heat of the moment and refrain from saying something we don't truly mean, or immediately apologize and clarify what we really meant to say. We help each other more often. And yes, we have a lot more sex.

. . . . .

But this section is not necessarily about increasing the amount of sex you have with your spouse. It is to increase the use of any form of intimacy that will let your partner know you're paying attention and that you care: playful touch, hand holding, back rubbing, extended hugs, forehead kisses, cuddling on the couch (yes, if you've been married for twenty or more years, you should still cuddle), a quick little butt smack while walking by each other in the kitchen, or a cat call from across the room when he/she is getting dressed. Any and all of these will increase the desire to be with each other more often. That is why I get so excited when couples sign up at our gym. I know that after a few weeks, they are going to become more intimate with one another because of what they are doing for themselves in the gym. It gets me fired up to help people lose weight, gain strength, feel more confident, start feeling sexy again, and, in turn, get that bed rocking every night after dinner.

. . . . .

What are you searching for in your connection with your significant other and the select few friends you're closest with? Joy? Satisfaction? Fulfillment? The same question is applicable in the context of what people search for in life. You'll hear so-called pundits argue that true happiness isn't obtainable. I roll my eyes every time I hear this argument between opposing sides. It's all obtainable. Even within your relationship, it's all obtainable. But in order to achieve those things, you have to understand that relationships of any kind sometimes conjure negative feelings, disagreements, or even arguments. If you open yourself up to this basic law of nature, it will allow you to experience the positive feelings that come with a relationship, as well. But you cannot ignore this simple truth about human interactions. You must embrace the negative feelings, and work through them without punishing yourself or your partner for having them. That hard work, in turn, allows for extreme happiness, and allows you to become more empathetic toward others. That's a tough boulder to shoulder. But not allowing negative feelings to stop you from feeling all of the positive ones is key. This might be a tough task to undertake, but it is essential in finding happiness within any kind of relationship.

But there must be some balance, as well. You cannot favor negative tendencies and then close yourself off to positive ones and vice versa. You're undermining your own happiness if you do this. You're creating your own suffering. Yes, you! If your spouse is doing the same thing, that certainly will not benefit you either, but your life, and what you envision for it, starts with you.

The Book of Joy: Lasting Happiness in a Changing World recounts a five day conversation between Archbishop Desmond Tutu and his Holiness the Dalai Lama. In the text, the Dalai Lama says, *"We create most of our suffering, so it should be logical that we also have the ability to create more joy. It simply depends on the attitudes, the perspectives, and the reactions we bring to situations and to our relationships with other people. When it comes to personal happiness there is a lot that we as individuals can do."*

I get it. If you're around your spouse for a few hours a day and he/she is a miserable cow, it's hard for you to be an optimistic butterfly. But before you blame someone else's behavior for your unhappiness, put yourself under the microscope and see if your negative feelings toward your spouse have created counterproductive communication habits. When is the last time you genuinely apologized to your partner for something you said or did? When is the last time you took it upon yourself to complete one of your partner's daily tasks, such as doing the laundry, cooking dinner, cleaning up dog poop, or taking out the trash? We are no longer living in the days when the man made the money and the woman kept the home. Both spouses should help each other with all aspects of keeping a house neat and orderly. Even if your spouse sucks at doing the laundry and doesn't fold clothes the same way you do, if he/she takes the initiative to do one of your chores, you shouldn't respond by berating an attempt to help around the house. Please, let that sink in. If you come home and your spouse is folding the laundry for the first time in a year, why on God's green Earth would your first inclination be to point out what he/she is doing incorrectly? Be freaking praiseworthy and thankful for the gesture! Crap, at least offer a hug and a kiss instead of saying, "It's about damn time!"

Here's where most of us are missing the boat. We don't just get unnecessarily annoyed with ourselves, but we are also too damn quick to get annoyed with our partners! It's very natural to feel some level of annoyance and frustration in a relationship, especially when you live with someone. Life isn't perfect, nor are our feelings, and when you build a life with someone, you won't agree on everything or do everything the same way. If you have expectations of always agreeing, you're setting your relationship up for failure. Welcome to real life. The perfect relationship does not exist. The huge differentiator between being a happy couple or not is understanding that feelings of occasional annoyance are natural and being okay with it[11]. But your partner isn't out to make your life hard or miserable. You need to learn what sets you off, and understand when and how it's appropriate to show these feelings. Not every emotion you feel needs to be expressed like a metaphorical tidal wave crashing into your partner's back while he/she is just laying on the beach, none the wiser until blindsided by its powerful force. I'm not talking about suppressing legitimately pressing issues or feelings,

---

[11] Start with a smile. Then, laugh it off. If your partner was gone, you'd miss those same annoyances.

but people tend to take little ripples in the water and stir them up until they've created unstoppable hurricanes that irreparably damage anything in their paths. Before you go and create the next tropical storm that appears as breaking news, ask yourself this: Are you really having a bad day, or did you just have a bad five minutes that you're milking all day? Calm down, Carl, and make sure your reaction appropriately matches the issue at hand.

· · · · ·

The irony of this chapter isn't lost on me. I've spent the previous seven encouraging you to prioritize these pillars to improve your own life. I've basically granted you permission to be self-centered, to fully focus on yourself and your goals. However, the most successful and fulfilled people are not self-made. People who have discovered true happiness and fulfillment have done so because they show kindness, compassion, and generosity toward other people. They've opened themselves up to experience genuine connections with other human beings.

For the first twenty-five years of my life, I was extremely selfish. I only focused on myself and my immediate family, and I thought I was happy. I certainly wasn't sad or depressed back then. But now, at the age of thirty, married with a daughter, and the owner of a gym that impacts the lives of people every single day, I can say that I am happier than I have ever been, and it's not because of what I have accomplished by myself. It's because of what all the people in my life are accomplishing despite potential roadblocks or struggles.

There is a huge difference between being self-centered, and being self-assured. Being self-centered impedes strong connections between humans, but being self-assured and recognizing your own accomplishments encourages others to do the same, promoting positivity and compassion that allows connections to grow.

So, although there is irony in discussing connections with other people in a book that promotes self-improvement, there is also perfect logic. With self-improvement comes self-assurance, with self-assurance comes positivity, and with positivity comes stronger interpersonal relationships.

· · · · ·

Somehow, the hardest pillar for me to write about, the one I avoided until the very end, became one of the longest chapters in this book. I realize that length does not indicate value, but I think it speaks to the complexity of this particular concept. Earlier chapters presented relatively cut and dry concepts, and the length of the chapters addressing them reflects that. We are human beings. One size does not fit all, and observing personal connections as though they exist on a continuum is a mistake that humans make all too often. So, as I look back through this chapter, which may seem fairly scatterbrained to some, I believe it is an accurate representation of how people need to work on this pillar: by engaging in metacognition and honestly evaluating how we behave in relationships, then seeking methods of making those behaviors better. In writing this chapter, I've done just that for myself. I hope that it may serve as a model for you to do the same.

Chapter Notes

Three Big Takeaways

1.

2.

3.

What do you currently do to build strong connections?

Do you currently view this pillar as a strength or a weakness?

What would you like to accomplish in regard to this pillar over the next 90 days?

12 months?

Are you committed? Can you do this?
P.S. The answer is, "Yes."

9 | THE CATALYST

I hate to be the bearer of bad news, but if you've read to this point in the book, and haven't changed even a single thing relating to the six pillars I've described, you are wasting your time. Even though I'm a huge fan of reading, you cannot just read about lifting weights and magically get better at lifting weights. You actually need to go and lift weights. In other words, you need to take action [12] in your efforts to better yourself. Not only must you take action, but it needs to be constant action. It needs to be enduring. It needs to be relentless.

If you don't, you will fail.

Exercise, food, sleep, personal development, stressors/media, and connection. Take control of those six pillars and you will reap the benefits of a better life. However, if you want to actually LIVE life, not just a better one, but your best life, your happiest life, there's one more thing that you need to take control of, and it's the foundation that these pillars are built upon: your mindset.

The way you talk to yourself, the way you perceive the outside world, the way you respond to both positive and

---

[12] Aka put your phone down, get off your ass, and actually go DO something productive that benefits you.

negative situations, what motivates your actions: all of these things define your mindset, and that mindset serves as the catalyst that allows these pillars to work together, ultimately resulting in changes far exceeding any that you've seen before.

. . . . .

While in the early stages of writing this book, I posted the following to Instagram and Facebook: "Stop adding fluff to your choices. The decisions and choices you make are binary. They are black or white, yes or no. There is no, 'Yes, but…' or 'I would have, but…' Make your choice, and stand by it. If something needs to change later on, then change it. But for right now, you either go and workout, or you don't. You either eat the cookie, or you don't. Stop adding fluff… fluff is just your excuses dressed up in a pretty bow."

After sharing that post, someone I have not spoken to since high school, over thirteen years ago, decided to come out of the woodwork and comment (Isn't it weird how that happens?). He wrote, "I don't think every choice is black and white. Actually, I think morality, or whatever a choice is based on, is on a spectrum. There's 180 degrees to my left, as well as to my right, and I can take either one of those paths."

I fully agree with what he said. "Any one of those paths." It doesn't matter if you view the world as black and white, or black, white, and 50 shades of gray. At the end of the day, you can only make one choice. It's true that we all have 180 degrees to the left, and 180 degrees to the right, but if you turn one degree to your left and draw a line long enough, guess what? You're really, really far away from where you originally would have ended up.

The binary way in which I view decision making may be unique to me, and if you disagree, that is fine. But allow me to clarify that I am not downplaying the complexity of the choices we have to make, nor the number of choices we have available to us. I'm referring to deciding "yes" or "no" on the majority of actions you're taking based on what you say you want. For example, say you take the plunge and start working out and eating better. After a week, you're feeling good and proud of yourself, but during week three, you have a cupcake. Don't body shame or ridicule yourself for eating one cupcake. Acknowledge what you did, and get back on track. You can work your way through some of your hiccups and still progress forward. What I mean when I say these types of decisions are black and white is this: you know the consequences of eating cupcakes, so if you continue to eat them, yet also keep telling people you want to lose weight, or complain that you're working hard and not seeing results, you're now adding fluff; you're saying you want a black shirt, but you keep buying all white. Not only are you making excuses, you're also lying to yourself and others.

· · · · ·

The following equation has appeared in numerous places, so I don't know who to credit for its creation, but I cannot discuss a positive decision making mindset without including it in this book.

$$E + R = O$$

Event + Response = Outcome

I'm not a math wizard, but it doesn't take one to understand what this equation clearly means: in life, events happen, and some of them are pretty shitty. The outcome of any event that occurs in your life is directly impacted by your response to it. Say, for example, that you are a gym owner. A probable "event" at some point in your career would be someone canceling a membership because he/she isn't receiving the expected results. It's pretty likely that your "response" will be driven by emotion. Maybe that emotion causes you to scold the client, pointing out that those "expected results" come from putting in hard work, not just attending two classes per week and sitting on the couch with any remaining free time. The outcome is that the client never comes back to your gym, and also tells everyone how rude you were, causing you to lose other potential clients.

Let's try it again.

The "event" is that someone cancels a gym membership because he/she isn't receiving the expected results. You respond by saying you are sorry to hear this news and you'd love to receive any input regarding how you could have improved the experience. You also send a card in the mail, thanking the client for contributing to your gym's community for the past twelve months. The outcome is that the now former client feels appreciated, and after two months of not being active, he/she decides to not only return to your gym, but also bring a spouse (since said client clearly read an incredibly motivating book about relentlessly pursuing a better life, and is working on both exercise and connections).

Same event, different responses, completely different outcomes.

Now, here is the key. You do NOT control most, if any, of the events that happen in your life. You do, however, control your initial reactions (usually emotional), and your actual responses (hopefully rational and action-oriented) to those events. So, with that being said, I reworked the equation to show what I feel actually occurs from a mathematical standpoint:

$$\frac{E}{2} + R^2 = O$$

(Event divided by 2) + Response squared = Outcome

    I truly believe that, no matter the level of the event that occurs in your life, you can diminish its value by dividing it by two (or four, or more, whatever it takes mathematically in your mind) while exponentially increasing the value of your response. This isn't a test. You're allowed to add shit in when needed in order to make it work! In my equation, your response has a much higher impact on determining the value of the outcome. You need to decide to lower the value of negative events[13] and place the majority, if not all, of your attention on your response to those negative events. Yes, there is a difference between spilling some coffee on your new blouse and getting a phone call that a loved one has passed away unexpectedly. But if you can't even properly handle spilling coffee, how are you going to push forward through

---

[13] I focus on negative events here, but if the event is positive, you need to leverage it by exponentially increasing its value ALONG with exponentially increasing your response. Again, it's your life, you can write the formula however you need to in order to gain the most positive outcome.

the grief of losing a loved one? Let's continue down the path of getting that phone call. Your initial responses will vary, but commonly this type of news is met with shock, anger, sadness, or even denial. Obviously, you cannot skip directly over these emotions, but the way you handle them will ultimately determine how smoothly and quickly you arrive at accepting the circumstances. The death of a loved one can push you into a deep depression from which you may never recover, or it can serve as a difficult, yet valuable lesson in overcoming adversity.

You need to understand that there is a strong correlation between your perception of the control you possess and what happens "for" you in your life. Notice, when I clarify that life happens for you, not to you, your perspective changes; you become empowered, in control. Positive action usually correlates with positive outcomes and vice versa (not always, but certainly more often than not). If you exercise and eat whole foods, you will become healthier. If you're nice and compassionate to others, you'll be well liked. If you can understand this correlation in the positive, then you can understand that the opposite may also be true. If you choose negative actions, then they will typically result in negative outcomes. Call this karma, call this fate, call this whatever you want, but the more good you sow for yourself, the more good you will reap. People say good things happen to good people, or that everything happens for a reason. I just like to think that the "reason" in that cliche quote is your chosen responses to events. Remember, events happen. You choose your response. And that response determines whether the outcome works in your favor or not.

·   ·   ·   ·   ·

   If you want to know how well you handle your responses to events, all you have to do is go for a drive. Road rage is quite the phenomenon. I'm not referring to the type of road rage that compels you to get out of your vehicle at a stoplight and bash the windows out of the car that just cut you off. I'm referring to road rage that most people view as minor: a quick horn honk, a middle finger, or an innocent shout of, "The speed limit is thirty five miles per hour, not thirty, you dumbass!" You think that every single person in the world should drive the way YOU drive: ten miles per hour OVER the speed limit. By doing so, you are not only reacting poorly to an event, but making something absolutely insignificant an event, too. And honestly, how big does your ego have to be to want everyone to drive the way you drive?

   Let's take all of the "fluff" away from that incident. You're driving ten miles per hour over the speed limit on a long, but straight back road. You catch up to someone driving five miles per hour under the speed limit, and you have ten more miles until your turn off. You start to get frustrated (while your child is in the back seat, mind you), and you start spouting off some word vomit. You are literally sitting in a rectangular metal box, screaming. And the person in front of you? He/she is sitting in a rectangular metal box, listening to Bon Jovi, and bellowing, "IT'S MY LIIIIFFFFFEEEEE, IT'S NOW OR NEVER," just living their best life! That person has no clue you're back there shouting all kinds of obscenities. And you? You just acted like a fool in front of your child. Not to mention you're now teaching an impressionable young person that it's appropriate to drive faster than other people and yell if they get in your way. That's all. Just over there setting a stellar example for your kids. And the "Parent of the Year Award" goes to…

If you can't even handle a Sunday driver, how are you going to respond to an inevitable setback in your relentless pursuit of a better you? You won't be able to. You have to change your mindset.

· · · · ·

Do you want to know what winners look like? Very few look like Lebron James or Tom Brady: tall, handsome, championship winning sports stars. I've heard before that a winner is someone who wakes up in the morning and makes the bed. I can see that, but it's not quite how I judge a winner. I make my bed every morning (Even though my wife would disagree with my definition of what "made" means). Making the bed isn't the measuring stick for being a winner; it might be the measuring stick for simple discipline, but not winning. Ask anyone at our gym, and he/she can tell you how I define a winner. A winner is someone who changes the toilet paper roll when it's empty. A winner is someone who puts the grocery cart back, even when it's cold and windy. People always want to change themselves, yet they don't even change the damn toilet paper in their own houses.

When it comes to making your bed, you return to it. You're only making it harder on yourself if you leave your side of the bed messy. But when you don't change the toilet paper roll or put your grocery cart back, not only are you leaving a job you started unfinished, you're putting that responsibility on someone else, and making that person's life slightly more difficult. That's what losers do. Although these may be minor examples, these situations overflow into other areas of your life. If you're working on a project with a few co-workers, you may leave parts of it incomplete since Jill has the ability to do it just as well as you, even though you told her you'd do it. You used up the last fifty sheets of paper in the printer, and, well, you're in a hurry, so you leave it empty, and when Dan tries to print off his proposal, he has to fill it up beforehand.

Changing the toilet paper can get annoying, but it's a part of the job. It's one of the many little tasks that no one talks about, but also says a lot about an individual. My close friends and I define discipline as doing the things you know you should do when you don't want to do them. Yes, you should make your bed. Yes, you should change the toilet paper and put your grocery cart back. And if you do those things most of the time, good. But what about the time you just legitimately forgot to make your bed? That doesn't make you a loser, a failure, or undisciplined. But the time you got out of your bed, acknowledged that it was a mess, and then told yourself it was okay to skip it? Now, that is being undisciplined. Those are the choices of someone taking a step down the path that strays away from the pursuit of a better self.

But, just as a winner doesn't necessarily look like Lebron James, the relentless pursuit of you isn't some intense, high energy, fast paced, hustle-until-you-die lifestyle. "Relentless" behavior can be associated with being aggressive, but that isn't necessarily always a bad thing. It's about being proactive: proactive toward all of life's little tasks, even the so-called "boring stuff." Always, every time, persistently. Be relentless in the mundane tasks of life, and you'll be relentless in achieving the extraordinary tasks, as well.

I'm sorry if discussing common daily tasks takes the "hype" out of the title *The Relentless Pursuit of You*, but it's the truth that you needed to hear. No one wants to hear about the bare basics and simple tasks in life. Why? Because it means that change is well within reach, but it requires work. Unfortunately, society wants to put talent and those who are born with a God-given ability to succeed up on a pedestal. But natural aptitude is not how most people who are successful have "made it." They've made it because they have a continual dedication to effectively completing the simple things in life, when the rest of society wants to lay back and have those things taken care of by someone else. The status quo wants to be told how hard life is so they can have an excuse as to why they didn't become as successful as they hoped. Winners don't make excuses. Winners persevere. Winners are relentless in pursuing success in all things, regardless of how big or how small.

· · · · ·

If I could look into the future and see one possible misinterpretation of this book, it is that readers mistake the idea of a "relentless pursuit" as an uncontrollable desire for more without ever being happy with their current state of affairs. That is certainly not what I'm promoting in this book. Understand that there is a dichotomy that exists when you set goals for yourself. Yes, you should be inspired to grow and develop, but at the same time, you should not become fixated only on achieving the end result of a goal, or the aspiration to continually acquire more wealth, possessions, or #gainz. Happiness is not on the other side of achievement, nor does fulfillment occur from merely accumulating desired titles or statuses. Focus on where you are in the moment, where you are in what Nick Saban[14] calls "the process," and the effort behind your pursuit. If you do this consistently and you do this well, you'll be more fulfilled than just focusing on the hype of the championship game.

If you want to relentlessly pursue a better you, the first step requires you to understand your current situation, no matter how dire or great it is. Understanding that you can grow, but also being perfectly okay with and loving yourself as you are today, is a fundamental component of having the right mindset to live a fulfilling life, both in this

---

[14] Six time NCAA Football Championship winning head coach

moment and in the future. I was told once that **if people are miserable today with what they have, they will be just as miserable when they have more of whatever it is they desire (money, fame, etc.).** The same mentality applies to how you interact in relationships. **If you can't love your partner when you're broke, how will you suddenly start loving that person when all of your bills are paid?** Don't get me wrong. I do love some of the finer things in life. Wanting material things isn't bad. What is bad, however, is when the desire for more material objects is greater than your desire to improve yourself, to be healthy, or to connect with others. Wanting more, more, more is detrimental when it comes at the cost of every other meaningful aspect of your life. I think it's safe to say that most people have come in contact with a miserable rich person. I certainly have! I wouldn't want that bank account if it meant having the same shitty attitude and depressing relationship.

    Even though the book *Good to Great* by Jim Collins is known for being one of the must-reads in the business world, he refers to a concept that really hits home for me on a personal level, and helped me understand the way I've viewed life as I've grown up. It was the first real book I read in adulthood, at the ripe old age of twenty-five, and sparked my interest in personal development and business growth. The concept Jim discusses is what's known as the

"Stockdale Paradox," named after United States Navy Admiral and Aviator James Stockdale, who was a Medal of Honor recipient and spent seven years as a prisoner of war. The concept instructs that *"you must retain faith that you will prevail in the end, regardless of the difficulties. And, at the same time, you must confront the most brutal facts of your current reality, whatever they might be."* This idea resonated with me long after I finished reading Collins's book. Up until that point in my life, I could never quite explain to people why I always continued forward, no matter the severity of the setbacks in my life. Having my final two consecutive high school football seasons cut short due to injuries didn't stop me from walking on to a national championship football team. Having a cash flow positive business go from something to nothing over the course of seven months didn't stop me from creating another, more successful business. Now, it all made sense. Sometimes close family and friends don't understand why I don't get worked up about setbacks all that much, or for all that long. It's because I believe that not much can truly destroy you or your life. I recognize that true suffering exists in this world, and I am not attempting to minimize the plights of those who have experienced that suffering. I'm very fortunate and grateful to have not had to experience incredible tribulations in my life. However, I also recognize that many people allow little setbacks to ruin their lives for far too long. It is my hope that you can address your current situation, no matter how troubled it is, and at the same time, believe that tomorrow will be better if you choose to make it better. Live your life as an optimistic realist.

. . . . .

While in the early stages of recreating your life's structural pillars and how they fit into your daily schedule, I want you to be strict, but, eventually, also being flexible becomes important. It's the person who understands the dichotomy between having a strict, yet flexible schedule who succeeds in the long term.

One day, you may oversleep by an extra twenty minutes, and have to forgo your morning stretches or reading, and that's okay. You might have an early flight before a long day of important meetings, so you prioritize rest. That's okay, as well. Try and slip in some semblance of your normal morning routine once you get to the airport and have a forty minute wait for your flight.

When looking at my daily schedule, I limit my important tasks of the day to no more than three items. There may be a few minor errands sprinkled throughout the day, but if I spend a little more time on an important task, I'll open my calendar up and move a minor errand to the next day or two. I find that limiting important daily tasks to less than three per day prevents me from getting overwhelmed or feeling rushed. That, in turn, allows me to put my full focus and energy into the limited tasks I've chosen for the day. I have taught myself to understand that my world will not fall apart if I don't do "all the things" today[15]. And lastly, once you prioritize your tasks, you have a plan of execution. One. Two. Three. And done.

    I am grateful that I currently have more freedom of choice over my schedule than most people. I've worked hard to achieve that, but it wasn't always the case. In a later chapter, I will lay out what my schedule looked like when I was still a teacher, husband, and father, working more than forty hours per week, along with how I implemented these pillars. My hope is that this shines some light on the fact that these pillars don't take an excessive amount of time, and that we can learn to engage in activities that address multiple pillars at once. For example, a client of mine, who is a single mom, once asked how to spend more time with her teenage daughter and continue to devote time to exercise and nutrition. My simple suggestion was that she start including her in prepping healthy dinners for the two

---

[15] Sometimes it's okay to let your dirty dishes sit for one more day, or let the dirty clothes basket get a little fuller if it means you spend more time on something of greater value in regard to your pillars, such as cuddling with your partner, playing with your child, walking your dogs, or meal prepping

of them. This would of course support her food pillar, but teaching her daughter how to cook would also build her connection (spending time together), personal development (learning a new skill), and stressors/media (staying off of social media during cooking time) pillars. How's that for killing two birds (or four, actually) with one stone?

Once you find some of the areas in your life that you are focusing too much or not enough time on, you'll be able to adjust, remove, and increase the priority level of various tasks on your new daily schedule. For example, I commend anyone who does volunteer work. Helping others is truly a selfless act, but at what cost? I recently went to coffee with a client of mine to discuss these six pillars as they relate to his life. He shared with me that he had spent 20 years of his life as a volunteer fire chief. Over those twenty years, he helped a lot of people in the local community. Mind you, he was also a full time career fire chief, husband, and father at the same time during which he was volunteering. Over this time, he let his health and relationships slip. With such a demanding schedule, that does not surprise me. He went on to tell me how difficult the decision to resign from his volunteer fire chief position was after his twentieth year. Want to know why he finally made the decision? He said, "I realized that I needed to gift time back to myself." Woah! I was blown away. I've never heard anyone use that phrase. I immediately wrote it down, starred it, and highlighted it so I would remember to come back to it later.

Giving to others is a lovely sentiment, but giving time back to yourself is possibly one of the most beautiful gifts anyone can either give or receive. It is something you both need and deserve. So, do it. Right now.

• • • • •

Maybe there are aspects of your life that currently seem out of whack, and you are seeking ways to find a "balance." Although your intentions are good, this idea of balance, especially work-life balance, is something I do not believe to be real. Work-life balance is a myth. Finding a perfect balance between all six of these important pillars is also unrealistic. Every day is different. Balance insinuates equality. You can't put your relationship and career on opposite sides of a balance scale and expect neither to weigh down the other. For example, I say I "don't work on the weekends." But, realistically, sometimes I do. I spend as much time as possible with my family every morning, every night, and every weekend, but every now and then, something needs to be taken care of, and Saturday night may be the only time it can be done. So, for those once in a while scenarios, I work on the weekend. It's not perfectly balanced.

When you think of balance, you may envision a tightrope walker slowly crossing a canyon, one thousand feet above the ground, entrusting his/her life entirely to nothing more than a thin rope. This daring individual seems to remain in perfect balance. But is that truly the case? Wait for the camera to zoom in on the feet. They aren't moving in a perfectly straight line. They are shifting from left and right. They are moving up and down. If the tightrope walker has a balance beam in his/her hands, either tip of the beam will rise or fall with every step. That's not perfect balance. Furthermore, this singular journey across this particular canyon is a micro event in the tightrope walker's life, just a snippet of a tightrope walking career that will inevitably be filled with a variety of similar situations. What we miss when we only focus on a micro event is the months or even years of walking on a rope only three feet above the ground, sometimes resulting in successfully meeting the finish line, but more often than not, falling off of the rope altogether. That's not balance. You shouldn't expect to always remain perfectly balanced when walking across this tightrope we call life. Sometimes you will fall off the side, and that's okay. You can always try again.

You can come up with your own opinions on what work-life balance means for you, but there is plenty of literature available to help you draw that conclusion. Take the Founder and CEO of Amazon, Jeff Bezos, for example. He has been quoted as telling new hires, and even executives at Amazon, that they should not strive for work-life balance: *"I get asked about work-life balance all the time. And my view is, that's a debilitating phrase because it implies there's a strict trade-off."* Instead of viewing work and life as a balancing act, Bezos believes you should view them as two integrated parts: "*It actually is a circle. It's not a balance.*" When you view work and life as working together, you can take your energy from one to the other like you're moving around the edges of a circle. You flow from one to the other, hopefully transferring the positive emotions gained from one directly to the other.

As human beings living in a fast-paced world, our priorities change daily, weekly, monthly, and annually. But within that tangled web we create for ourselves, the true challenge is maintaining some control over our schedules. You hear it all of the time: "I'm just so busy!" But being busy doesn't mean you're being productive. Being busy doesn't mean you're progressing, growing, or improving. Being busy doesn't mean you're being smart. You think all of these things that make you "busy" dictate your schedule, but you have more control than you have allowed yourself to believe. You're just making stupid decisions regarding how to use your time. It's okay to admit it, but I hope it hasn't taken you up until this moment in the book to realize you're wasting a large majority of your day doing things that neither help you improve yourself, nor bring you joy.

In Chapter 10, we will dissect your day into fifteen minute segments, but start thinking about this now. If you sleep seven hours per night, and work eight hours per day, that leaves you with nine unencumbered hours each day! WHAT ARE YOU EVEN DOING, BRO?! Let's go a step further and say that you actually work ten hours per day. You'd still have seven extra hours to do everything else. That's a whole other "work day" you could be using to devote to yourself! But what's frustrating is that quite a few people reading this book either won't finish reading (they won't see this section since they stopped way too early), or they won't take the time to audit their schedules and face the reality that they waste more time than they thought.

In order to win the day, you don't have to perfectly fulfill all of these pillars throughout every single twenty-four hour cycle. It begins by writing out what your schedule would look like on a pretty damn good day. And here's the kicker: you probably won't follow that schedule verbatim tomorrow, or next week, or even every day a year from now. As I mentioned in the introduction of this book, the goal is to negotiate with yourself. Always remember what I tell my clients: pretend there are two entirely separate versions of you. The current you, the you reading this book, who is breathing and living today. And then the future you, the you you'll be in a few months or years if you win 90% of the negotiations with yourself today for your future self. Don't take the number 90% too seriously, though. Even if you only meet 50% or 75% of the expectations of your new schedule, it's still a lot better than 0%. You still win. But, the only way to meet your future self is to win the majority of your daily negotiations. Yes, you love how donuts taste. But if you lose that negotiation every day or every other day, you're not going to meet your future self, who finally understands that donuts don't bring you happiness, and who has stopped eating them because the taste lasts less than a minute and it's not worth it. That's how you win the day. You must win the small daily negotiations with yourself.

· · · · ·

Now that we've established that a good part of your schedule is in your control, let's talk about what's out of your control. Basically, everything else: everyone who may or may not be judging you, everyone you compare yourself to, strangers you see on social media, the global political issues scattered across the television, the things that have happened in your past. All of those things are out of your control. You're attempting to control all of the wrong things.

So what is it that you should try to control? Your procrastination. Your neglect. Your ego. The negative behavior you're voluntarily participating in every single day. Control that. Take ownership of failed attempts to control these things in the past because we both know you wouldn't be reading this book if they had been successful. We have all experienced that level of failure, but if you can't accept that as fact, you will not be able to move on, and you will continue to fail. Good or bad, it's on you[16]. Wage war with your decisions. Take a stand against doing the things you know are not making your life better, including how you talk to yourself.

Imagine your friend comes to you and admits that he/she doesn't feel good enough anymore. This friend has gained a few pounds, tried working out for the last week to no avail, is constantly fighting with a spouse, and just "sucks at life." How quick are you to point out a whole list

---

[16] *It's On You* was actually the working title of this book when I first started writing, but after a few weeks, I felt I needed something stronger to hammer my point home. However, I still love this line because, well, it *is* on you.

of positive characteristics you see in that friend in the hopes of providing uplifting support? What if your son or daughter comes walking off of the soccer field for the first time, and despite how proud you feel, the first comment out of his/her mouth is, "Mom, I suck compared to all of the other kids." How do you react? With loving support and an explanation about time, patience, and hard work. You reiterate how proud you are, and that you're there to help with improving throughout the season.

Then, the very next day, you go to the gym and are in a group with fifteen other people whose ages range from twenty to sixty, and waistlines from zero to twenty-four. Upon finishing class, you shake your head in frustration and walk to your car, feeling defeated because you moved so slowly, couldn't lift the same weight as the lady next to you, and everyone probably thinks you're pathetic. No. Actually, that's not what anyone thinks about you. In fact, they probably aren't thinking about you at all, so why is that the thing you're fixating on?! Working out and contributing to your exercise pillar is a daily victory, no matter if you think it went well or not. If you get to the gym or do something active for the day, you've won a small battle. So, give yourself a personal high five and some self-love for God's sake!

As a gym owner, I see this often. A new client comes in (we'll call her Susie), and she is nervous, timid, uncoordinated, and unhealthy. She is my favorite type of client because I know after only a few workouts, she will see improvements in not only how she controls her body, but also her confidence in being able to work out regularly with the support of our coaches. Fast-forward a couple of months and Susie is jumping rope for the first time since grade school, jumping on a twenty inch box for the first time in her life, and can deadlift the same amount as she used to weigh. I say "used to weigh" because most clients typically lose so much fat that they need to buy new workout clothes. She has made incredible progress in a short amount of time! Then, I see her walk over to the pull up rig after class and try a pull up for the first time. She barely moves off of the ground. Her chin drops, eyes go to the floor, and she shakes her head. Sounds sad and unrealistic, doesn't it? No. It happens. All. Of. The. Time. So, I walk over and Susie says, "I just want to get my first pull up so bad!" And, being a supportive, but realistic coach, I reply, "That's a great goal and we can help you with that, but remember six months ago when you couldn't even press that barbell over your head for three reps? But in today's workout you pressed that same barbell overhead with added weights on it for over fifty reps. You've come a long way, and you should be proud. Don't let the goal of getting a pull up make you forget how much you can actually do nowadays compared to when you started. I like that you want to keep progressing and you have set some new goals, but when you started, you were just hoping to become the person you are today."

Let's fast forward another few months. Susie has finally gotten her first pull up! Amazing! Then, a workout comes up where there are ten pull ups per round. She got her first pull up the other day, so she should be able to get a couple in the workout, right? Or at least that's what she thinks. So, she starts the workout with a short run, and with her heart rate elevated, she can't get beyond a fourth pull up, try as she might. Her chin drops, eyes go to the floor, and she shakes her head. Sounds sad and unrealistic, doesn't it? No. It happens. All. Of. The. Time. And again, I have to remind Susie of the talk we had a few months prior, when all she wanted was her first pull up. And today, she got four in a workout with an elevated heart rate! I remind clients often that there is zero positive that comes out of negative self-talk, and fixating on the things you can't do instead of the progress you've made (no matter how big or small) will eventually cause you to lose motivation altogether.

Why is this the case? Why are we so hard on ourselves? Well, is it because you've read a book about relentlessly pursuing you, and that means you always have to strive for bigger, better goals? No. I want you to celebrate your victories. I want you to be able to put your life, your abilities, your progress, and the timelines required to improve yourself in a perspective that is realistic. We've allowed society to tell us that if we celebrate our victories, that makes us self-centered and egotistical, so we just keep our mouths shut when we accomplish things that make us proud. No. Celebrate what you can do and what you've accomplished! Those who mind don't matter and those who matter don't mind. And when you encounter an obstacle or a challenge you aren't quite ready to face yet, instead of dropping your chin and shaking your head, lift it up and smile. You now have something to strive for, an opportunity to improve and grow.

Positive self-talk is fine and dandy, but it makes no difference if you can't identify when you're being too hard on yourself and find a way to pause and correct your behavior. You may not always have someone with you who recognizes your negative body language and calls you out for your obvious self-doubt, so it is up to you to realize how hurtful those self-deprecating thoughts are to your mindset and your progress toward achieving a goal. You have to become aware of when those thoughts occur and take responsibility for actively working to change them. Try to think back to the last time you were abusing yourself inside of your head, especially when other people were around. Maybe it was during a group workout, or at the office around your co-workers. Now, imagine your thoughts were projected through a loudspeaker so all of those people around you could hear how you talk to yourself. Would you be proud of what they get to hear? Let's go a step further. You're working out with your best friend, Amy. You start to have some toxic, negative self-talk inside that head of yours. This time, I want you to imagine that, instead of simply thinking poorly of your own workout, you look at Amy, and offer similar criticism about her workout. "Hey, Amy! Why are you so damn slow and weak? You really aren't cut out for this whole exercise thing. Do you know that? Oh, by the way, your new workout pants make your legs look fat, and I hate your hair color." It looks like you just lost a friend, you big bully.

If you are a parent, it's likely that your child getting bullied is one of your worst fears. Our hearts break thinking about children who get bullied, and we get infuriated at the bullies, their parents, and their teachers for allowing it to happen. Then, we turn around, and in essence, bully ourselves. We beat ourselves up over things we've done, things we've allowed others to do to us, and things that haven't even happened yet.

In *12 Rules for Life: An Antidote to Chaos*, clinical psychologist and professor Dr. Jordan Peterson's second rule is to "*treat yourself like someone you are responsible for helping.*" While mentioning how easy it is to believe that people are arrogant, egotistical, and only looking out for themselves, he makes it clear that this is not the case for many people: "*They have the opposite problem: they shoulder intolerable burdens of self-disgust, self-contempt, shame and self-consciousness. Thus, instead of narcissistically inflating their own importance, they don't value themselves at all, and they don't take care of themselves with attention and skill. It seems that people often don't really believe that they deserve the best care, personally speaking. They are excruciatingly aware of their own faults and inadequacies, real and exaggerated, and ashamed and doubtful of their own value. They believe that other people shouldn't suffer, and they will work diligently and altruistically to help them alleviate it. They extend the same courtesy even to the animals they are acquainted with--but not so easily to themselves.*"

This is exactly what this book has been about: self-care, not self-sacrifice. It's not selfish to work toward improving yourself, especially if it means that you will, in turn, serve others. I think back to all of the amazing mothers and fathers I've worked with over the years, who, after having children, let their health slip. They helped raise amazing children, but to what end? Could they have raised even better children, harder working children, more understanding children, healthier children, if they themselves would have worked hard to be healthy, physically and mentally, using the pillars described in this book? I think the answer is, "Yes." And that concept is something I will continue to reference as I, myself, raise a family.

. . . . .

Now, it's on you to finally make the decision to be unrelenting, to take the first step. Regardless of what you've done with your life up until this point, you are made for more. You are the only one who will determine how your life will end up. You control your future. Think of that person you'll be a year from now, five years from now, ten years from now. I can't wait for you to meet that person. I cannot wait for you to look in the mirror at some point in the future and come face to face with the person who decided enough was enough, the person who decided to take ownership of his/her life and finally become relentless in the pursuit of improvement. That person is going to be you. I'm excited for you and I cannot wait to hear your story. Start now. Put your hand on your heart. Close your eyes and tell yourself that you've got this. Because you do. You have this beating heart inside of you that wants more for yourself and your life. Smile and wipe away that tear that just rolled down your face, Crystal. Let's go.

10 | JOURNAL

Let's get to work. First, you're going to audit your average day by breaking it down into fifteen minute increments. If you don't know what your average day looks like or how much time you spend on each pillar, then fill it out through the next day or so. I suggest writing in pencil because it may surprise you to see what you're actually doing… or not doing.

Remember, most people overestimate what they can do in a day, but underestimate what they can do in a year. Focus on getting as detailed as possible when outlining your day. While reading through this book, you may have found areas of strength and areas of weakness, but right now, you need to have the most accurate self-assessment you've ever had. You may not be happy with what you realize about yourself, but that is okay. You need to know where you really are before you know where you can go. Additionally, put some extra attention on your food pillar. In my experience, when I ask, "What's your food pillar look like? What do you eat?" most reply with, "I eat pretty well." And in all honesty, they don't. You may be inclined to keep a separate sheet of paper, or download a food tracking app to get a real analysis of what you are eating on a daily basis.

Follow the directions below. I have personal examples further down.

The Pillars - Look at your notes from the end of each chapter, and use them to accurately describe what you're currently doing for each pillar, how often, and whether each is a strength or weakness.

External
Exercise →
_____
_____

Food →
_____
_____

Sleep →
_____
_____

Internal
Personal Development →
_____
_____

Stressors / Media →
_____
_____

Connection →
_____
_____

Using the blank worksheet following my example, indicate what pillars you are addressing at any given time of the day.

Use the following indicators: Food (F), Exercise (E), Sleep (S), Personal Development (P), Stressors/Media (M), Connection (C), and Work (W).

The following is an example of what my worksheet currently looks like:

Example Day for Shawn

4:00am S	10:30am WM	5:00pm C
4:15am S	10:45am WM	5:15pm C
4:30am S	11:00am WM	5:30pm FC
4:45am S	11:15am WM	5:45pm FC
5:00am S	11:30am WM	6:00pm C
5:15am S	11:45am WM	6:15pm C
5:30am FE	12:00pm PD	6:30pm C
5:45am FE	12:15pm PD	6:45pm C
6:00am FPD	12:30pm PD	7:00pm C
6:15am FPD	12:45pm PD	7:15pm C
6:30am C	1:00pm PD	7:30pm PD
6:45am C	1:15pm PD	7:45pm PD
7:00am C	1:30pm FPD	8:00pm C
7:15am C	1:45pm PD	8:15pm C
7:30am C	2:00pm PD	8:30pm C
7:45am C	2:15pm PD	8:45pm C
8:00am EC	2:30pm PD	9:00pm C
8:15am EC	2:45pm WC	9:15pm S
8:30am EC	3:00pm WC	9:30pm S
8:45am EC	3:15pm WC	9:45pm S
9:00am E	3:30pm WC	10:00pm S
9:15am E	3:45pm WC	10:15pm S
9:30am W	4:00pm WC	10:30pm S
9:45am W	4:15pm WC	10:45pm S
10:00am W	4:30pm WC	11:00pm S
10:15am W	4:45pm WC	11:15pm S

Your Current Schedule

4:00am ____	10:30am ____	5:00pm ____
4:15am ____	10:45am ____	5:15pm ____
4:30am ____	11:00am ____	5:30pm ____
4:45am ____	11:15am ____	5:45pm ____
5:00am ____	11:30am ____	6:00pm ____
5:15am ____	11:45am ____	6:15pm ____
5:30am ____	12:00pm ____	6:30pm ____
5:45am ____	12:15pm ____	6:45pm ____
6:00am ____	12:30pm ____	7:00pm ____
6:15am ____	12:45pm ____	7:15pm ____
6:30am ____	1:00pm ____	7:30pm ____
6:45am ____	1:15pm ____	7:45pm ____
7:00am ____	1:30pm ____	8:00pm ____
7:15am ____	1:45pm ____	8:15pm ____
7:30am ____	2:00pm ____	8:30pm ____
7:45am ____	2:15pm ____	8:45pm ____
8:00am ____	2:30pm ____	9:00pm ____
8:15am ____	2:45pm ____	9:15pm ____
8:30am ____	3:00pm ____	9:30pm ____
8:45am ____	3:15pm ____	9:45pm ____
9:00am ____	3:30pm ____	10:00pm ____
9:15am ____	3:45pm ____	10:15pm ____
9:30am ____	4:00pm ____	10:30pm ____
9:45am ____	4:15pm ____	10:45pm ____
10:00am ____	4:30pm ____	11:00pm ____
10:15am ____	4:45pm ____	11:15pm ____

Example Day for a Full-Time Working Schedule

4:00am S	10:30am W	5:00pm C
4:15am S	10:45am WC	5:15pm C
4:30am S	11:00am WC	5:30pm FC
4:45am F	11:15am WC	5:45pm FC
5:00am E	11:30am FPD	6:00pm C
5:15am E	11:45am FPD	6:15pm C
5:30am E	12:00pm WC	6:30pm C
5:45am E	12:15pm WC	6:45pm C
6:00am E	12:30pm WC	7:00pm C
6:15am PD	12:45pm WC	7:15pm C
6:30am C	1:00pm W	7:30pm PD
6:45am C	1:15pm W	7:45pm PD
7:00am C	1:30pm W	8:00pm C
7:15am C	1:45pm WC	8:15pm C
7:30am C	2:00pm WC	8:30pm C
7:45am C	2:15pm W	8:45pm C
8:00am C	2:30pm W	9:00pm C
8:15am C	2:45pm W	9:15pm S
8:30am W	3:00pm W	9:30pm S
8:45am W	3:15pm W	9:45pm S
9:00am WC	3:30pm PDM	10:00pm S
9:15am WC	3:45pm PDM	10:15pm S
9:30am WC	4:00pm PDM	10:30pm S
9:45am WC	4:15pm PDM	10:45pm S
10:00am W	4:30pm C	11:00pm S
10:15am W	4:45pm C	11:15pm S

Your New "Pretty Damn Good Day" Schedule

Describe what you'd like to accomplish in regard to each pillar, and label your new schedule worksheet below accordingly.

External
Exercise →
_____
_____

Food →
_____
_____

Sleep →
_____
_____

Internal
Personal Development →
_____
_____

Stressors / Media →
_____
_____

Connection →
_____
_____

4:00am ____	10:30am ____	5:00pm ____
4:15am ____	10:45am ____	5:15pm ____
4:30am ____	11:00am ____	5:30pm ____
4:45am ____	11:15am ____	5:45pm ____
5:00am ____	11:30am ____	6:00pm ____
5:15am ____	11:45am ____	6:15pm ____
5:30am ____	12:00pm ____	6:30pm ____
5:45am ____	12:15pm ____	6:45pm ____
6:00am ____	12:30pm ____	7:00pm ____
6:15am ____	12:45pm ____	7:15pm ____
6:30am ____	1:00pm ____	7:30pm ____
6:45am ____	1:15pm ____	7:45pm ____
7:00am ____	1:30pm ____	8:00pm ____
7:15am ____	1:45pm ____	8:15pm ____
7:30am ____	2:00pm ____	8:30pm ____
7:45am ____	2:15pm ____	8:45pm ____
8:00am ____	2:30pm ____	9:00pm ____
8:15am ____	2:45pm ____	9:15pm ____
8:30am ____	3:00pm ____	9:30pm ____
8:45am ____	3:15pm ____	9:45pm ____
9:00am ____	3:30pm ____	10:00pm ____
9:15am ____	3:45pm ____	10:15pm ____
9:30am ____	4:00pm ____	10:30pm ____
9:45am ____	4:15pm ____	10:45pm ____
10:00am ____	4:30pm ____	11:00pm ____
10:15am ____	4:45pm ____	11:15pm ____

ACKNOWLEDGEMENTS

To think that it was only a short five years ago that I was sitting on the floor, back against my bed, crying at the thought of my first business failing, and having to start all over again. It was my wife, Cait Rider, who found me like that, picked me up, and said that it would all work out if we just took another step forward. And now here I am, writing the acknowledgements to a book that hopefully helps at least one person take back his/her life. I could not and would not have done this if it hadn't been for the support of my wife. Cait, thank you for giving me the drive and time to complete this project. You are an incredible person and an even better wife and mother.

I want to recognize my editor, Crystal Gage, who has been a client at our gym for over five years now. She is an AP English Teacher at John Handley High School. When I asked if she'd be interested in helping me edit my book for simple grammatical errors, she jumped at the opportunity. But little did I know what she could actually do. After getting the edits for the first chapter back, I was blown away at the value she brought to the table. It has been a fun process to watch her execute her craft. I get to coach her on a regular basis in the gym, but seeing her coach me through the writing process was a very rewarding flip of the script. Her ability to rewrite, reorganize, and clarify my thoughts while keeping my voice has been invaluable. This book would not be what it is if it wasn't for her. So, Crystal, thank you.

To the team members at our gym, thank you for your patience as I took a step away to focus on getting this message out. I have learned so much from each of you, and it is my hope that our clients realize that this book is a collection of all of our thoughts on how to improve lives.

And to the clients at our gym, thank you for giving me the courage and inspiration to share what we believe in at Shenandoah.Fit. Without your support, I would not have had the confidence to write this book.

Finally, I'd like to thank all of the authors and influencers who have shared their experiences with me through books, videos, and podcasts: Jim Collins, Ryan Holiday, Marcus Aurelius, Dalai Lama, Desmond Tutu, Jocko Willink, Leif Babin, Gary Vaynerchuk, Carol Dweck, Angela Duckworth, Jordan Peterson, Phil Knight, Ed Mylett, Lewis Howes, Andy Frisella, and Tony Robbins.

REFERENCES

Chapter 2: The Pillars

Dweck, C. S. (2006). *Mindset: The New Psychology of Success*. New York, NY: Random House.

Roosevelt, T. (2009). *The Autobiography of Theodore Roosevelt*. Seven Treasures Publications.

Chapter 4: Food

Glassman, G. (2002, October 1). What is Fitness? Retrieved from https://journal.crossfit.com/article/what-is-fitness

Willink, J., & Babin, L. (2017). *Extreme Ownership: How U.S. Navy SEALs Lead and Win* (2nd ed.). New York, NY: St. Martin's Press.

Chapter 6: Personal Development

Duckworth, A. (2018). *Grit: The Power of Passion and Perseverance*. New York, NY: Scribner.

MasterClass (2019). Retrieved from https://www.masterclass.com/

Wikipedia. (2019, April 3). Personal development. Retrieved from https://en.wikipedia.org/wiki/Personal_development?scrlybrkr=47c3ffa7

Chapter 7: Stressors / Media
Aurelius, M. (2014). *Meditations*. Edinburgh, UK: Black & White Classics.

Chapter 8: Connection
Bstan-'dzin-rgya-mtsho, D.L., Tutu, D., & Abrams, D.C. (2016). *The Book of Joy: Lasting Happiness in a Changing World*. New York, NY: Avery.

Wikipedia. (2019, May 15). Dunbar's number. Retrieved from https://en.wikipedia.org/wiki/Dunbar%27s_number

Chapter 9: The Catalyst
Bernard, Z. (2019, January 9). Jeff Bezos' advice to Amazon employees is to stop aiming for work-life 'balance' — here's what you should strive for instead. Retrieved from https://www.businessinsider.com/jeff-bezo-advice-to-amazon-employees-dont-aim-for-work-life-balance-its-a-circle-2018-4

Collins, J. (2001). *Good to Great: Why Some Companies Make the Leap and Others Don't*. New York, NY: HarperCollins Publishers Inc.

Peterson, J.B. (2018). *12 Rules for Life: An Antidote to Chaos*. Toronto: Random House Canada.

Made in the USA
Middletown, DE
03 June 2019